MORTALITY AMONGST ILLICIT DRUG USERS

Over the past 40 years the rate of illicit drug use worldwide has risen dramatically, and with it the number of deaths reported among drug-using populations. What are the clinical, ethical, and psychopathological implications of these deaths? In this book, Shane Darke and his team provide the first full, synthetic review of the epidemiology, causes, prevalence, demography, and associated risk factors of illicit-drug-related mortality. In addition, they examine and evaluate interventions to reduce these deaths. The major causes of death among illicit drug users are overdose, disease, suicide, and trauma. Each is independently examined. This is an important book for all clinicians and policy-markers involved in issues relating to illicit drug use.

SHANE DARKE is Associate Professor at the National Drug and Alcohol Research Centre at the University of New South Wales. He is also Australasian Regional Editor of *Addiction* and an associate editor of *Drug and Alcohol Dependence*.

LOUISA DEGENHARDT is Senior Lecturer at the National Drug and Alcohol Research Centre at the University of New South Wales. She is also Senior Investigator of the Illicit Drug Reporting System and the National Illicit Drug Indicators Project.

RICHARD MATTICK is Professor and Director of the National Drug and Alcohol Research Centre at the University of New South Wales. He is a Member of the Editorial Boards of *Drug and Alcohol Review*, and the *Cochrane Review Group of Drugs and Alcohol*.

INTERNATIONAL RESEARCH MONOGRAPHS IN THE ADDICTIONS (IRMA)

Series Editor
Professor Griffith Edwards
National Addiction Centre
Institute of Psychiatry, London

Volumes in this series present important research from major centres around the world on the basic sciences, both biological and behavioural, that have a bearing on the addictions. They also address the clinical and public health applications of such research. The series will cover alcohol, illicit drugs, psychotropics, and tobacco. It is an important resource for clinicians, researchers, and policy-makers.

Also in this series:

Cannabis Dependence: Its Nature, Consequences and Treatment
Roger A. Roffman and Robert S. Stephens
ISBN 0 521 81447 2

Gambling as an Addictive Behaviour: Control, Harm Minimisation, Treatment and Prevention
Mark Dickerson and John O'Connor
ISBN 0 52184701 X

Circles of Recovery: Self-help Organizations for Addictions
Keith N. Humphreys
ISBN 0 521 79299 0

Treatment Matching in Alcoholism
Thomas F. Babor and Frances K. Del Boca
ISBN 0 521 65112 3

A Community Reinforcement Approach to Addiction Treatment
Robert J. Meyers and William R. Miller
ISBN 0 521 77107 2

Cannabis and Cognitive Functioning
Nadia Solowij
ISBN 0 521 159114 7

Alcohol and the Community: A Systems Approach to Prevention
Harold D. Holder
ISBN 0 521 59187 2

MORTALITY AMONGST ILLICIT DRUG USERS: EPIDEMIOLOGY, CAUSES, AND INTERVENTION

SHANE DARKE, LOUISA DEGENHARDT & RICHARD MATTICK

National Drug and Alcohol Research Centre
University of New South Wales
Australia

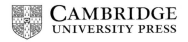
CAMBRIDGE
UNIVERSITY PRESS

CAMBRIDGE UNIVERSITY PRESS
Cambridge, New York, Melbourne, Madrid, Cape Town, Singapore, Sao Paulo

Cambridge University Press
The Edinburgh Building, Cambridge CB2 2RU, UK
Published in the United States of America by Cambridge University Press, New York

www.cambridge.org
Information on this title: www.cambridge.org/9780521855068

Printed in the United Kingdom at the University Press, Cambridge

A catalogue record for this publication is available from the British Library

Library of Congress Cataloguing in Publication data

ISBN-13 978-0-521-85506-8 hardback
ISBN-10 0-521-85506-3 hardback

Cambridge University Press has no responsibility for the persistence
or accuracy of URLs for external or third-party Internet web sites
referred to in this publication, and does not guarantee that any
content on such web sites is, or will remain, accurate or appropriate.

Contents

Acknowledgements

This work was made possible through the funding of the Australian Government Department of Health and Ageing. The authors wish to thank Eva Congreve for her tireless help in conducting literature searches and tracking down references. We also wish to thank Professor Wayne Hall for his invaluable comments on drafts, and Anna Williamson for her forensic eye for detail in proof reading, and her excellent comments on drafts.

List of tables

1

Why illicit drug-related deaths matter

1.1 Introduction

Over the course of the past 40 years, the use of illicit drugs has increased dramatically in developed nations. Over this period there have been substantial increases in the use of cannabis, opioids, cocaine, amphetamine, and, more recently, amphetamine-like substances such as MDMA ("ecstasy") (cf. Chapter 2). While the initial increase in illicit drug use occurred within developed nations, recent years have seen large increases in illicit drug use in the developing world. In particular, since the 1990s there have been substantial increases in rates of drug use and drug-related problems in countries such as China, India, and the Republics of the former Soviet Union (Degenhardt et al., 2004a; United Nations Office for Drug Control, 2005).

Clearly, the use of illicit drugs has become an issue worldwide, although the nature of the problem may well vary from nation to nation. In some nations cocaine may be the primary focus, whilst in others opiates may dominate clinical concern. A natural corollary of any increase in the use of illicit substances of any sort, however, is an increase in rates of illicit drug-related death. The use of illicit drugs carries risks for morbidity and mortality, either directly related to the drug itself (e.g. overdose) or as a consequence of such use (e.g. intoxicated driving). As will be seen repeatedly throughout this book, rates of death amongst illicit drug users are substantially higher than those seen amongst the non-drug using population (cf. Chapter 3).

It is undeniable that both drug use and drug-related mortality have increased. The question posed in this chapter, however, is does this matter? Are there ethical reasons why this should be a concern to society or, indeed, for devoting a book to examining these deaths? It could be argued, for example, that such deaths are by nature self-inflicted, and that the deaths of illicit drug users may well be beneficial to society. After all, it could be said that nobody forces illicit drug users to expose themselves to risk by taking drugs, and the reduction in crime and disease represented by their deaths may constitute a net gain to society. Whilst the authors of this book may not concur with this view, the issue of why such deaths are a matter for public concern is one that does require addressing, before embarking upon a detailed exploration of these deaths and the means to reduce them. There are a number of ethical and utilitarian arguments that emphasise the importance of drug-related death to society. Broadly speaking, these fall into the following areas: (i) ethical responsibility to prevent avoidable death, (ii) the costs of such deaths to society, (iii) the natural history of drug use, and (iv) the impact of such deaths on the families of drug users.

1.2   Why illicit drug-related deaths matter

1.2.1   *Ethical responsibility to prevent avoidable death*

The first thing to note in any discussion of whether illicit drug-related mortality matters is the extent of the problem. As will be more fully discussed in Chapter 3, it was estimated that in 2000 alone there were approximately 200,000 deaths worldwide attributable to illicit drug use (Degenhardt et al., 2004a). This figure is undoubtedly a conservative underestimate of the true level of mortality (cf. Chapter 3). As would be expected, given the epidemiology of illicit drug use (cf. Chapter 2), the majority of deaths occur amongst younger people, with the average age at death being approximately 30 years.

As a general rule, the prevention of premature death is uncontroversial. Few would argue that premature death due to leukaemia, for example, does not matter, or that the victims in some way deserved to die. Drug use, however, raises passions that are rarely seen when discussing death due to other causes. Unlike a disease brought on by some external factors, death due to drug use is essentially self-inflicted. The ethical responsibility thus falls upon the user, who has taken the decision to use and, typically, to continue to use illicit drugs. The distinction between drug use mortality and other forms of mortality is thus between what could be termed a "lifestyle choice" compared to death due to extraneous causes beyond the control of the individual.

As with so many appealing dichotomies, however, a simple contrast between a self-chosen pathway to death and other forms of mortality does not withstand close scrutiny. There is a clear implicit assumption of unrestricted free will in the assertion that drug-use behaviours are self-determined. Leaving the issue of free will versus determinism aside, the literature demonstrates clear precursors for increased risk of illicit drug use and substance dependence (cf. Chapter 2). In particular, the development of problematic illicit drug use has been strongly associated with what has been referred to as a "shattered childhood" (Rossow & Lauritzen, 2001). This term includes a general clinical picture of parental psychopathology, parental drug and alcohol problems, early loss of parents, and, most importantly, childhood sexual and physical abuse (Rossow & Lauritzen, 2001). The development of drug-dependence problems is thus not a random occurrence, but is strongly associated with a set of factors likely to increase psychological distress and, not surprisingly, problematic drug use. Consistent with this picture of a "shattered childhood", levels of serious psychopathology such as major depression are extremely high amongst dependent illicit drug users (Darke & Ross, 1997a; Dinwiddie et al., 1992; Lynskey et al., 2004; Teesson et al., 2005). The majority of problematic drug users thus come from backgrounds that increase their risk of serious psychopathology and of dependent drug use. Much of this drug use may, in fact, be seen as attempts to self-medicate distressing effect.

The second point to raise concerning the "choice" of a drug using lifestyle is that, as will be seen in later chapters, the majority of drug-related fatalities occur amongst dependent drug users. Substance dependence is, of course, a well-recognised psychiatric diagnosis, defined in both the Diagnostic and Statistical Manual of Mental Disorders (DSM-IV) (American Psychiatric Association, 2000) and the International Classification of Diseases (ICD-10) (World Health Organization, 1993). The syndrome includes both physical (e.g. withdrawal) and psychological (e.g. salience of the substance in the person's life) symptoms. Like many other psychiatric disorders (e.g. major depression, anxiety disorders, schizophrenia) drug dependence is strongly associated with substantially increased risk of premature death (Harris & Barraclough, 1998). Broadly speaking, the core feature of substance dependence is a loss of control over use of the substance in question. The person may be physically dependent on the drug, experiencing drug tolerance and withdrawal symptoms, and continue to use despite repeated efforts at abstinence. The point here is that, by definition, to invoke drug use as a choice when the person had been diagnosed as having lost control over their drug use is absurd. There are clear psychosocial factors that heighten the risk of illicit drug use and, once dependence has developed, to speak of choice makes little sense.

Moreover, the typical onset of illicit drug use, and of drug dependence, occurs in the teenage years (Chen & Kandel, 1995; Degenhardt et al., 2000; Kandel et al., 1992), *prior* to the person becoming an adult deemed ethically or legally responsible for their own behaviours. Legally, societies do not hold children to be sufficiently developed cognitively or ethically to make informed, free choices of great magnitude. The use of illicit drugs, clearly, is a behaviour that carries enormous implications for health and welfare. To hold children or adolescents ethically responsible for a self-chosen pathway to death, particularly when adverse events in childhood so strongly predict such behaviours, is inconsistent and absurd. While the person may die an adult, the dependence that leads to this death, typically, was acquired as a minor.

Even if we assume that drug-related deaths are self-inflicted, however, it is unclear how they could be distinguished from other fatalities that *are* universally deemed worthy of clinical interest and intervention. The self-inflicted death *par excellence*, clearly, is death by suicide. Even if it is assumed that drug use, and dependent drug use, is a freely chosen pathway to mortality, drawing a distinction between death due to drug use and death due to suicide is difficult. If killing oneself, or attempting to kill oneself, is a matter for clinical and societal concern, then death from drug use is surely a similar matter for concern. No logical distinction can be drawn. Of course, problematic drug use might well be seen as a form of prolonged self-destruction, further blurring distinctions between drug-related mortality and suicide. Certainly as noted previously, there are high rates of depression and suicidal ideation amongst dependent drug users. In fact, suicide itself is a major cause of death amongst illicit drug users, as will be discussed at length in Chapter 7.

The problem of distinguishing self-inflicted deaths from other deaths that are worthy of intervention, however, extends far beyond the prime example of suicide. Let us take the cases of licit drug-related death, due to tobacco- or alcohol-related disease. To be consistent, these too would have to be deemed unworthy of intervention, as the use of these drugs was also a freely chosen lifestyle choice. So too would deaths resulting from motor vehicle accidents attributable to excessive speed (a freely chosen behaviour) or obesity-related illness due to excessive eating. The argument is never consistently applied, yet no logical or ethical distinction can be drawn between mortality due to illicit drug use and other deaths that *are* deemed worthy of concern.

1.2.2   Costs to society

The second broad issue to consider is the cost to society of drug-related mortality. As noted above, it could be argued that drug users constitute a substantial cost to society primarily through crime and disease. Given these costs, the attrition through death of illicit drug users may well be seen as a reduction of the burden that drugs impose upon society.

There is no doubt that drug use, and dependent drug use in particular, does place a substantial cost burden upon societies. In particular, there is a strong association between dependent drug use and crime (Flynn et al., 2003; Gossop et al., 1998; Kaye et al., 1998). It is important to note that this association, specifically, is between drug use crimes committed by dependent drug users to acquire money to purchase drugs, such as robbery or drug dealing. Importantly, however, the frequency of acquisitive crime has been demonstrated to co-vary with the frequency of illicit drug use. As the frequency of drug use declines, so also does the rate of acquisitive crime (Flynn et al., 2003; Gossop et al., 1999; Hser et al., 1998; Simpson et al., 1997). In fact, one of the major societal benefits of drug-treatment programmes is that criminal behaviours decline markedly as a result of such treatment.

In addition to crime, illicit drug use, and injecting drug use in particular, is strongly associated with disease and disease transmission. The sharing of used injecting equipment is a major transmission factor for human immunodeficiency virus (HIV), hepatitis C virus (HCV), and hepatitis B virus (HBV) (Karch, 2002). There are a range of other pathologies associated with drug use, including cardiovascular disease, pulmonary disease, renal complications, and neuropathology (Cherubin & Sapira, 1993; Karch, 2002). It is beyond question that regular illicit drug users are in poorer health than the non-drug using population, due to the complications of drug use. As with crime, however, the health of illicit drug users improves substantially after entering drug-treatment programmes (Gossop et al., 2002a).

While there are clearly substantial costs associated with illicit drug use, the deaths of large numbers of drug users also impose a substantial cost upon society. As noted above, the average age of illicit drug user deaths is around 30 years (Chapter 3). Given the relatively young age of such deaths, there is considerable lost productivity due to the truncated lifespan. It was recently calculated that in the year 2000 alone, nearly 7 million Disability Adjusted Life Years (DALYs), a measure of lost life and lost productive life, were attributable to death from illicit drug use (Degenhardt et al., 2004a). As will be discussed in Chapter 3, this is in all probability a substantial underestimate of the lost life and productivity incurred by illicit drug use.

The view that illicit drug users place a continuous burden upon society is predicated upon an assumption that problematic drug users always commit crime, and place burdens upon the health system. As noted above, however, sharp declines in criminality and improvement in both physical and psychological health are associated with drug-treatment programmes. Naturally, then, the burden imposed by criminal behaviours and poor health will decline, while levels of social functioning improve. Problematic drug users may be a burden whilst using drugs, but this burden is ameliorated by treatment and declines with their drug use.

The above discussion primarily relates to dependent drug users. Typically, the picture of high levels of crime and extremely poor health presented above primarily pertains to a long-term heroin or cocaine user (Cherubin & Sapira, 1993; Karch, 2002). Whilst many deaths occur among unemployed, long-term opioid or cocaine users, as will be seen in subsequent chapters, a proportion of illicit drug use deaths occur amongst recreational users of cannabis or designer amphetamine-like drugs (e.g. MDMA "ecstasy") (Chapter 4). Cannabis, for example, is strongly associated with motor vehicle accidents (cf. Chapter 7), whilst deaths occurring from the use of drugs such as MDMA may result from hyperthermia or cardiac arrest (cf. Chapter 4). The psychosocial profile of such users is completely different from that of the regular, dependent opioid or cocaine user. These are typically employed, recreational users who are at low risk of serious diseases such as HIV or HCV. These are, in effect, typical young members of society. To characterise such productive young persons as a societal burden clearly would be absurd.

1.2.3   Natural history of drug use

The next point to consider, the natural history of drug use, follows on from the previous discussion on costs to society. As discussed above, illicit drug use typically commences in the mid-teenage years. Importantly, it peaks in the 20–30-year age group, and declines sharply in older age groups (Chen & Kandel, 1995; Degenhardt et al., 2000; Kandel et al., 1992). The natural history of illicit drug use is thus skewed towards the younger years. The point here is that the label "illicit drug user" is not an immutable lifetime description, but may refer to a relatively brief period. A person may well use illicit drugs during their 20s, but most will cease to do so in later years. The highest risk of illicit drug use, and of thus of mortality, is focussed over a relatively brief period in the person's life. If this high-risk period can be navigated safely, then the person may well cease to be an illicit drug user and cease to impose any illicit drug-related costs upon society. Even if we accept a view that illicit drug users are in some sense unworthy of concern, these same people may well cease to be illicit drug users after a relatively short period.

Dependent drug use, and opioid dependence in particular, may of course persist for substantially longer than the patterns described above (Hser et al., 2001). Even dependent opioid use, however, is cyclical in nature. Opioid users go through periods of use, followed by periods of treatment and abstinence (Darke et al., 2005c; Flynn et al., 2003; Hser et al., 2001). Many dependent users may be seen to mature out of drug use, although this may take considerable time. As noted above, it is incontrovertible that drug-treatment programmes produce substantial improvements in the psychosocial profile of dependent drug users. As is the case with recreational drug users, there is a natural history associated with dependent drug use. A dependent drug user may be a high-risk person who imposes a societal burden. They may not, however, remain a dependent drug user, or continue to impose such a burden.

1.2.4   Families of drug users

Finally, we must consider the impact of illicit drug use deaths upon the families of these users. It is beyond question that the loss of loved ones through drug use matters greatly to the families of drug users. In considering whether drug use mortality is a legitimate matter for concern, the drug user must not be seen in isolation. The death of a drug user does not only affect the user themselves, but also those surrounding them. While it could be argued that the death was self-inflicted, this in no way applies to the anguish of relatives, partners, and friends of the deceased drug user. The effects upon the loved ones of deceased drug users are something that clearly must be considered when examining the impact of drug-related death. Apart from the lost societal productivity of the decedents themselves, drug deaths impose large burdens upon the families, and partners of deceased drug users.

Even if we were to restrict the argument to a strict utilitarian approach, and confine our analyses to the impacts upon broader society, there are good reasons to be concerned about familial loss through drug use. The most salient issue here clearly concerns the children of drug users. Early parental loss is associated with increased risk of the development of subsequent psychopathology, as well as increased risk of drug dependence and of suicide (Fergusson & Lynskey, 1995; Rossow & Lauritzen, 2001). One major advantage in keeping illicit drug users alive is that such actions may well reduce the costs to society of illicit drug use and drug-related death among the next generation. As noted above, most illicit drug use occurs over a relatively brief period in a person's life. If this period can be lived through, this may have substantial benefits for the families of drug users, both currently and in the future.

1.3   What do we need to know about illicit drug-related mortality?

Ultimately, whether illicit drug user deaths matter or not is a question that must be decided by the reader. If they do not matter, then there is nothing further to say. If we do accept that high rates mortality amongst illicit drug users is a matter of concern, however, then what do we need to know about such deaths? First, we clearly need to understand the epidemiology of illicit drug use (Chapter 2). What are the drugs being used, and by whom? Second, what are the mortality rates associated with illicit drug use, and amongst whom are such deaths occurring (Chapter 3)? Third, what is causing such deaths, and how do these causes differ by substance (Chapters 4–7)? Finally, how can the rates of illicit drug user mortality be reduced (Chapter 8)? The ensuing chapters of this book will examine the epidemiology of illicit drug use, the epidemiology of drug-related death, the causes and factors associated with such deaths, and the efficacy of attempts to reduce drug-related mortality.

1.4   Summary

In summary, there are good reasons, apart from compassion for the victims, to regard illicit drug user mortality as a serious matter of public concern. Rates of illicit drug-related death have dramatically increased worldwide since the 1960s, and represent a major cause of death amongst younger people. Arguments that death due to illicit drug use is essentially self-inflicted and therefore not a matter for societal concern do not stand up to close scrutiny. There are well-delineated psychosocial factors that engender regular illicit drug use, and most drug-related fatalities occur amongst drug dependent individuals who have lost control of their drug use.

   Whilst the use of illicit drugs imposes substantial costs upon societies, there are also substantial costs incurred through lost years of productivity from what are primarily deaths among young people. It is also the case that drug users do not necessarily remain drug users, and may move beyond drug use to make substantial contributions to society. Finally, drug users do not live in isolation. Drug-related mortality impacts upon the families of decedents, and increases the risks of serious psychopathology, drug dependence, and suicide amongst the children of deceased users.

Key points: Summary of why illicit drug use deaths matter

- Rates of illicit drug use and drug-related deaths have dramatically increased in the developed world since the 1960s, and in developing nations since the 1990s.
- Deaths due to illicit drug use are not due to a self-inflicted, freely chosen lifestyle. There are well-delineated psychosocial factors that engender regular illicit drug use.
- Most drug-related fatalities occur amongst drug dependent individuals who have lost control of their drug use. Moreover, drug use and dependence typically commences prior to the person having become an adult.
- The use of illicit drugs imposes substantial costs upon societies. There are also substantial costs to society, however, incurred through lost years of productivity from deaths among young people.
- Drug users do not necessarily remain drug users, and may move beyond drug use to make substantial contributions to society.
- Drug users do not live in isolation. Drug-related mortality impacts upon the families of decedents.

2

The global epidemiology of illicit drug use

2.1 Introduction

In this chapter, we outline the global epidemiology of illicit drug use. Illicit drug use includes the non-medical use of a variety of drugs that are prohibited by international law. These drugs include methamphetamine, amphetamine, MDMA (ecstasy), cannabis, cocaine, heroin, and other opioids. Table 2.1 briefly outlines the major drug classes. In order to estimate mortality attributable to illicit drug use, we need to define which drugs we are speaking about, and consider the relative prevalence of their use.

2.2 Drug use or drug use problems?

Most people who use psychoactive substances do so without experiencing any problems related to their use, but some do develop problems (Anthony et al.,

Table 2.1. Selected drugs and their actions

Drug type	Actions
Amphetamine type stimulants (ATS)	A class of sympathomimetic amines with powerful stimulant action on the central nervous system (CNS).
Cannabis	Generic term for psychoactive preparations derived from the *Cannabis sativa* plant (e.g. marijuana, hashish, hash oil).
Cocaine	An alkaloid CNS-stimulant drug derived from the coca plant.
MDMA	3,4-Methylenedioxymethamphetamine. Synthetic drug used as a (ecstasy) stimulant.
Opioids	Generic term applied to derivatives from the opium poppy, their synthetic analogues, and compounds synthesised in the body, which act upon the opioid receptors in the brain (e.g. heroin, opium, methadone). They have the capacity to relieve pain and produce a sense of euphoria, as well as to cause stupor, coma, and respiratory depression.

1994). The conceptualisation and measurement of these problems has undergone considerable change over the past three decades, with the emergence of the concept of a substance "dependence syndrome", influenced by Edwards and colleagues' work on alcohol dependence (Edwards & Gross, 1976). In 1977, Edwards and colleagues suggested that alcohol *dependence* could be thought of as a cluster of symptoms that were distinguishable from alcohol-related problems occurring in heavy drinkers (Edwards et al., 1977). The concept of a dependence syndrome has since been extended to substances such as cannabis, tobacco, amphetamines, opioids, and sedatives. Another category of problematic substance use has also been developed: the concept of substance *abuse*. This was developed in an attempt to classify persons who experienced clinically significant problems associated with their substance use, but who were not using the substance in a dependent manner.

The most recent operationalisation of the substance abuse and dependence syndromes is DSM-IV (American Psychiatric Association, 2000). DSM-IV Substance Abuse criteria require a pattern of substance use that causes clinically significant distress or impairment. DSM-IV Substance Dependence criteria require a cluster of three or more indicators (of a possible seven) that a person continues to use the substance despite significant substance-related problems (American Psychiatric Association, 2000). These include tolerance, withdrawal, indicators of impaired control over use, use despite problems, and the reduction of activities not related to substance use.

The World Health Organization (WHO), following the International Classification of Disease (ICD-10), defines problem drug use as "harmful drug use" and "drug dependence". Harmful drug use is defined by clear evidence that substance use is responsible for physical (e.g. organ damage) and psychological harm (e.g. drug-induced psychosis). Drug dependence, as defined in ICD-10, requires the presence of three or more indicators of drug dependence (World Health Organization, 1993). These include a strong desire to take the substance, impaired control over use of the substance, a withdrawal syndrome on ceasing or reducing use, tolerance to the effects of the drug, requiring larger doses to achieve the desired psychological effect, a disproportionate amount of the user's time being spent obtaining, using and recovering from drug use, and the user continuing to take drugs despite associated problems. These problems must have been experienced at some time during the previous year for at least 1 month.

The United Nations Drug Control Programme (UNDCP) identifies "problem drugs" based on "the extent to which use of a certain drug leads to treatment demand, emergency room visits (often due to overdose), drug-related morbidity (including HIV/AIDS, hepatitis, etc.), mortality and other drug-related social ills"

(United Nations Drug Control Programme, 2000). It is important to note that in the majority of cases, it is problematic or dependent patterns of drug use, rather than occasional or experimental use, that best predict mortality from drug use.

2.3   How common is illicit drug use?

The use of drugs for non-medical purposes appears to be increasing in many parts of the world (United Nations Office for Drug Control, 2005). One of its defining features, its illegality, makes it difficult to quantify how many drug users there are (European Monitoring Centre for Drugs and Drug Addiction, 1997, 1999b). This is for a number of reasons. First, illicit drug-using individuals are "hidden" and may be difficult to identify. Second, even if drug users can be located and interviewed, they may attempt to conceal their drug use. Third, prevalence estimates vary with the method used and assumptions made. Data provided by the United Nations Drug Control Programme do not have the same reliability as large-scale household surveys of the type generally conducted in developed countries. Unfortunately, the expense of conducting such surveys makes their use in developing countries unfeasible.

There are no well-tested and widely accepted "gold standard" methods for producing credible estimates of the number of people who make up the "hidden population" of illicit drug users (Hartnoll, 1997). The preferred strategy is to look for convergence in estimates produced by a variety of different methods (European Monitoring Centre for Drugs and Drug Addiction, 1997, 1999b). These methods are of two broad types, *direct* and *indirect*. Direct estimation methods attempt to estimate the number of illicit drug users in representative samples of the population. Indirect estimation methods attempt to use information from known populations of illicit drug users (such as those who have died of opioid overdoses) to estimate the size of the hidden population.

Prevalence data reported in peer-reviewed literature are scarce and often unrepresentative. There has been even less research on the epidemiology of *substance use disorders* in the general population than there has on *substance use*. Some exceptions are the US Epidemiological Catchment Area (ECA) study and the US National Comorbidity Study (NCS), which found that the most commonly used substances were also the most commonly *misused* substances (Anthony & Helzer, 1991; Anthony et al., 1994). The same was also found in the more recent Australian National Survey of Mental Health and Well-Being (Hall et al., 1999c).

It is important to remember that there is strong evidence (principally from developed countries) that few drug users use one drug exclusively (Darke & Hall,

1995; Darke & Ross, 1997; Dinwiddie et al., 1996; Gossop et al., 2002; Hubbard et al., 1997; Klee et al., 1990; Ross & Darke, 2000). Rather, most users nominate a drug of choice but regularly use a wide range of substances.

2.3.1 Cannabis

Cannabis is the most widely used illicit drug in most developed and many developing countries (Hall et al., 1999b). There are notable differences in the prevalence of cannabis use across developed countries. Rates appear higher in the UK, some western European countries, the USA, Canada, and Australia (with adult lifetime rates of use that can reach around 35–40%) than in countries such as Romania and Belgium (where rates are around 1–7%) (Hall et al., 2001). The more limited data available from developing countries in Africa, the Caribbean, Asia, and South America suggest that rates of cannabis use are much lower in these countries than in Europe and English-speaking countries (Hall et al., 2001, 1999b). In all countries, rates of past year use are highest among young adults.

2.3.2 Amphetamine-type stimulants

Increases have been noted in recent years in the market for amphetamine-type stimulants (ATS) in many countries (United Nations Office of Drug Control). Production and consumption of ATS appear to have increased considerably in recent years, notably around the Pacific Rim – North America, South-East Asia, and Oceania (United Nations Office for Drug Control, 2005). Many countries in these regions have noted the increased use of crystal methamphetamine, first in the Philippines, Korea, Taiwan, and Japan (Laidler & Morgan, 1997; Matsumoto et al., 2000; Shaw, 1999; Suwaki, 1991), and later in the US (Laidler & Morgan, 1997; Morgan & Beck, 1997; National Drug Intelligence Centre, 2003). In recent years, crystal methamphetamine use has been increasing in availability in areas of Oceania (Farrell et al., 2002; McKetin et al., 2005a, b; Topp et al., 2002; Wilkins, 2002).

The United Nations estimated that there were 26 million methamphetamine or amphetamine users globally in 2003 (United Nations Office for Drug Control, 2004). In European countries, lifetime prevalence of amphetamine use typically ranges from 0.1% to 6%, although rates are higher in the UK (up to 12%) (European Monitoring Centre for Drugs and Drug Addiction, 2005). In the USA, the prevalence of amphetamine use was estimated at 8.3% (Substance Abuse and Mental Health Services Administration, 2005).

Similar increases also appear to have occurred for "ecstasy", the name for tablets sold purporting to contain MDMA (United Nations Office for Drug Control, 2005). Ecstasy use has traditionally been concentrated in developed countries in North America, Europe, and Australia (United Nations Office for Drug Control, 2005). In Australia, ecstasy use among the general population has increased from 1% in 1988, to 7.4% in 2004 (Australian Institute of Health and Welfare, 2005). Indeed, ecstasy is now the second most widely used illicit drug in Australia among young adults aged 20–29 years. This is consistent with the trends seen in Europe, with ecstasy becoming more commonly used than amphetamines (European Monitoring Centre for Drugs and Drug Addiction, 2005).

2.3.3   Cocaine

Cocaine use is largely restricted to the Americas, which is not surprising given that production of cocaine occurs almost exclusively in that region (United Nations Office for Drug Control, 2005). It has been estimated that there are 14 million cocaine users globally, of which two-thirds are found in these regions. Worldwide, the prevalence of cocaine use has been estimated at 0.3% (United Nations Office for Drug Control, 2005), but cocaine use has historically been significantly higher than this in the USA (Johnston et al., 2003), which experi-enced a so-called "epidemic" of cocaine use (particularly in "crack" cocaine form) during the 1980s (Agar, 2003; Miech et al., 2005). Although crack cocaine use has declined in the USA since that time (Bowling, 1999), the prevalence of cocaine use remains more prevalent in that country than in comparable countries such as Australia (Johnston et al., 2003). In the USA in 2004, 14% of those aged 12 years or older reported lifetime use of cocaine use, and 2.4% reported hav-ing used it during the previous 12 months (Substance Abuse and Mental Health Services Administration, 2005).

Recent years may have seen an increase in the availability and use of cocaine in Europe, and increases in the use of "crack" cocaine (Home Office, 2004). Recent population surveys estimate that between 0.5% and 6% of the European population have tried cocaine, with rates in Italy (4.6%), Spain (4.9%), and the UK (6.8%) being higher than elsewhere in Europe (European Monitoring Centre for Drugs and Drug Addiction, 2005).

2.3.4   Heroin and other opioids

The prevalence of opioid use is relatively low in comparison with other illicit drugs. Estimates produced by the United Nations suggest that globally, just over 15 million people had used opioids in the previous year (United Nations Office for Drug Control, 2004). This corresponded to approximately 0.4% of the global population aged between 15 and 64 years. Of these people, just over 9 million were estimated to use heroin, or approximately 0.2% of the global population aged 15 to 64 years (United Nations Office for Drug Control, 2004).

According to the UNODC, over half of the world's opioid users are to be found in the Asian countries surrounding Afghanistan and Myanmar, the two biggest opium cultivating countries (United Nations Office for Drug Control, 2004). Four million opioid users are estimated to be found in Europe (mostly in Eastern Europe). North and South America combined account for about 2.5 million opioid users, and Oceania (which includes Australia) has been estimated to have 0.1 million users. Both Europe and Oceania have a prevalence of opioid use higher than the global average: 0.75% and 0.5% of the population aged 15 to 64, respectively (United Nations Office for Drug Control, 2004).

There have been recent changes in opioid use globally. Use appears to be stable or declining in Western Europe, East and South-East Asia, Pakistan, and some Central Asian countries. China has experienced considerable increases in the extent of heroin use over the past decade, with the number of registered "addicts" reaching 1 million in 2003, a 15-fold increase since 1990 (United Nations Office for Drug Control, 2005).

There have been particularly marked decreases in problems related to heroin use in Australia since 2001 (Degenhardt et al., 2005b, c, e), and possibly in the number of regular heroin users (Degenhardt et al., 2004b, 2005c), as a result of a marked reduction in heroin supply and apparently sustained changes in the structure and extent of heroin trafficking into the country.

2.4 Risk factors for illicit drug use

Simple prevalence estimates of the proportion of the population that have *ever* used an illicit drug are likely to be associated with a low average risk of mortality. This is so because a single occasion of use and infrequent use are the most common patterns of reported use in population surveys, and these patterns are associated with only a small increase in mortality.

There are some global demographic factors that strongly predict illicit drug use. In general, males are more likely than females to use most psychoactive substances (Greenfield & O'Leary, 1999; Johnston et al., 2000a, b; Kandel, 1991). There are indications, however, that this gender difference in rates of use may be diminishing in more recent birth cohorts. While marked gender differences exist in the prevalence of substance use among older birth cohorts, these differences became smaller in more recent birth cohorts (Degenhardt et al., 2000). Illicit drug users are also likely to be married/de facto than those who have not used illicit drugs (Kandel, 1991; Kandel et al., 1997; Warner et al., 1995).

Substance use (particularly illicit substance use, but also alcohol and tobacco use) is strongly associated with a person's age. Young people are by far the most likely age group to report using psychoactive substances within the past year (Bachman et al., 1997; Makkai & McAllister, 1998). Recent use (e.g. past year) typically declines in adulthood, reflecting the adoption of roles such as child-rearing, marriage, and employment (Bachman et al., 1997).

One hypothesis to explain why some people seem more likely to develop problematic substance use is that they inherit an increased susceptibility (*vulnerability*) to the development of such problems. Substance use disorders are likely to cluster within families. Researchers have attempted to develop models of vulnerability to substance use disorders, in which vulnerability is the product of genetic and/or environmental factors. Research with twins suggests that there is a significant genetic component (*heritability*) that increases the likelihood of dependence on a range of substances. Twin studies have produced estimates of the heritability of cannabis abuse and dependence (ranging from 62% to 79%) (Kendler & Prescott, 1998a; Tsuang et al., 1998), and also for dependence upon heroin, sedatives, and stimulants (Kendler & Prescott, 1998b; Tsuang et al., 1996, 1998). The exact nature of these genetic vulnerabilities is not known. Thus far, there have been no single candidate genes discovered which are directly related to substance abuse (Altman et al., 1996). It is likely that genetic influences involve multiple genes or the incomplete expression or function of several genes that influence how drugs are metabolised and how rewarding their effects are (Kendler, 1999; Schuckit, 1999).

There are several social and environmental factors that have been strongly related to substance use and substance use disorders. These are in keeping with the findings of twin studies showing that while there is a strong genetic component accounting for vulnerability to substance dependence, there is also a substantial *environmental* component (e.g. Kendler & Prescott, 1998a, b; Kendler et al., 1999). A number of these factors will be outlined below.

There is abundant evidence that people who engage in antisocial behaviour are more likely to have, or develop, substance use problems. Adolescents with conduct disorders are significantly more likely to develop substance use disorders than those without such conduct problems (Cicchetti & Rogosch, 1999; Gittelman et al., 1985). In general, it appears that the earlier, more varied and more serious a child's antisocial behaviour, the more likely it will be continued into adulthood, with substance misuse considered one of these antisocial behaviours (Costello et al., 1999; Robins, 1978). Furthermore, children or young people with anxiety or depressive symptoms are more likely to begin substance use at an earlier age, and more likely to develop substance use problems (Cicchetti & Rogosch, 1999; Costello et al., 1999; Henry et al., 1993; Loeber et al., 1999).

The peer environment also has a large influence on substance use behaviours. Substance use usually begins with peers, and peer attitudes to substance use have been shown to be highly predictive of adolescent substance use (Fergusson & Horwood, 1997; Hoefler et al., 1999; Newcomb et al., 1986). This may be because those who use substances are more likely to choose to spend time with other people who use such substances. There is, however, no direct evidence on the influence of peers on the development, or maintenance, of substance *dependence* (Institute of Medicine, 1996).

Families also have a strong effect upon the likelihood that people will develop substance use problems (Hawkins et al., 1992; Lynskey et al., 1998). This occurs in a number of ways. First, modelling of substance use by parents and other family members has been shown to affect adolescent substance use behaviour. For example, parental substance use has been associated with the initiation of alcohol and cannabis use (Hawkins et al., 1992), while older brothers' substance use and attitudes towards substance use have been associated with younger brothers' substance use (Brook et al., 1988). Second, there is evidence that if parents hold permissive attitudes towards the use of specific substances by their children, their children will be more likely to use such substances (Hawkins et al., 1992). Third, the nature of family relationships has an effect upon the likelihood that adolescents will develop problematic substance use. The risk of substance misuse is higher if there is family discord, poor or inconsistent behavioural management by parents, or low levels of bonding within the family (Hawkins et al., 1992).

The socio-cultural background of a person will also affect the likelihood that they develop substance use problems. There are clear links between social disadvantage and poorer global health outcomes (Graham & Power, 2004; Wilkinson & Marmot, 2003). More particularly, there are strong links of disadvantage with substance use, which suggest increased vulnerability of the disadvantaged to the initiation of substance use, and thus be exposed to its associated problems (Anthony et al., 1994; Hawkins et al., 1992; Kandel et al., 1997). Disadvantage may be conceptualised at three levels: individual disadvantage, family disadvantage, and community disadvantage. At the level of individual disadvantage, lower socioeconomic individuals are more likely to have problematic use across a range of substances, including tobacco, alcohol, and illicit drugs (Anthony et al., 1994; Hawkins et al., 1992, Hemmingsson et al., 1997; Muntaner et al., 1998). More specifically, markers for individual disadvantage such as unemployment and lower educational levels have been associated with the use of illicit drugs such as cannabis, amphetamines, and heroin (Institute of Medicine, 1996; Kandel, 1991; Kandel et al., 1997; Lynskey & Hall, 2000; Warner et al., 1995).

When considering the disadvantage of an individual and potential for illicit drug use, childhood family disadvantage must also be taken into consideration (Bradley & Corwyn, 2002; Graham & Power, 2004). Lower parental socio-economic status has been associated with a number of risk factors for the development of substance use and dependence such as childhood abuse, childhood neglect, depression, and hopelessness (Bradley & Corwyn, 2002; Galea et al., 2004; Graham & Power, 2004; Poulton et al., 2002). The more specific subsequent effects of such childhood factors upon mortality due to suicide amongst drug users are discussed in a later section (Chapter 6).

Finally, community disadvantage is associated with a range of health and social problems (Bobashev & Anthony, 1998; Galea et al., 2004; Petronis & Anthony, 2003; Weatherburn & Lind, 2001). In particular, disadvantaged communities have higher rates of initiation into alcohol and illicit drug use, and of substance use problems (Bobashev & Anthony, 1998; Fergusson & Horwood, 1997; Galea et al., 2004; Hawkins et al., 1992; Institute of Medicine, 1996; Petronis & Anthony, 2003; Weatherburn & Lind, 2001). For instance, the incidence of fatal opioid and cocaine overdose, a clear marker of use of these drugs, has been associated with the poverty of a district (Marzuk et al., 1997). Impoverished social environments tend to have high rates of crime, delinquency, and substance availability. In the case of the disadvantaged community, we see a clustering of the disadvantages discussed above with limited educational opportunities, lower levels of employment, and higher levels of stress upon individuals and families.

2.5   Summary

Cannabis is the most commonly used illicit drug in many societies. Stimulant drugs such as amphetamines, ecstasy, and cocaine are typically the next most commonly used drugs. Opioid drugs are the least commonly used drugs worldwide.

Substance use has been consistently linked to a number of social and demographic characteristics, with males, younger persons, unemployed persons, those with less education, those who are not married, and those from lower socioeconomic backgrounds all more likely to report licit and illicit substance use. Disadvantage at the individual, family, and community level all increase the likelihood of substance use. In general, these same factors have also been related to an increased risk of problematic substance use.

A multitude of theories have been proposed to explain why some people develop problematic substance use. Genetic factors appear to play a part: twin studies indicate these components have a significant role in developing dependence upon the most commonly used substances. There is also consistent evidence that a range of environmental factors will increase the likelihood of problematic substance use. These include economic disadvantage, family conflict, modelling of substance use or parents' permissive attitudes towards substance use, as well as childhood conduct disorder and emotional problems.

There are a number of approaches to explain why some people become problematic substance users. Each level of explanation (biological, psychological, socio-cultural) has been supported by empirical research. These different levels, however, remain to be integrated into a more comprehensive model of addiction.

Key points: Summary of illicit drug use epidemiology

- There is a clinical distinction between substance use, substance abuse, and substance dependence.
- Cannabis is the most commonly used illicit drug in many societies.
- Stimulant drugs such as amphetamines, ecstasy, and cocaine are typically the next most commonly used drugs.
- Opioid drugs are the least commonly used illicit drugs worldwide.
- Substance use has been linked to social and demographic characteristics: being male, younger age, unemployment, less education, unmarried, lower socioeconomic background.
- Genetic factors appear to play a significant role in developing dependence upon the most commonly used substances.
- Environmental factors will increase the likelihood of problematic substance use: family conflict, modelling of substance use, permissive parental attitudes towards substance use, childhood conduct disorder, emotional problems.
- Individual, family, and community disadvantage all increase the likelihood of illicit drug use and dependence.

3

Mortality amongst illicit drug users

3.1 Introduction

In this chapter we examine the epidemiology of illicit drug-related death. Specifically, this chapter presents rates of mortality amongst illicit drug users from all causes, the demography of cases, and the associated risk factors. As any discussion of illicit drug-related mortality must necessarily discuss the issues surrounding the estimation of drug-related mortality, they are examined first. Rates of death due to specific causes will be examined in subsequent chapters, as will the specific factors associated with these causes.

3.2 Problems in estimating mortality

A number of problems arise when attempting to estimate global mortality attributable to illicit drug use (cf. Degenhardt et al., 2004a). Part of the problem arises from the very fact that the drugs in question are illicit, and that these deaths thus occur amongst "hidden" populations. Whilst a death may be attributable to illicit drug use, the use of these drugs may well have been concealed by the individual. As such, the link to illicit drug use may not be formally recognised as the cause of death, or as a factor associated with the death. A good example is the completed suicide of an illicit drug user, an issue addressed in detail in a later chapter. If the suicide method is by means of an illicit drug overdose, then the death will be clearly attributable to illicit drug use. If, however, the suicide is performed by means that do not involve drugs (e.g. hanging), association of the death with illicit drug use may not be made. The decedent may be an illicit drug user, the death may be due to depression associated with drug use, but unless the illicit drug using status of the individual is known, such an attribution will not occur. Reported death rates amongst hidden populations are thus, in all likelihood, underestimates.

It is also obvious that the quality of official statistics on the prevalence of illicit drug use, and of illicit drug-related mortality, will vary enormously from country to country. A wealthy, first world country is far more likely to have the resources and infrastructure to devote to collecting official statistics on mortality and its specific causes than would a poorer nation. Estimates of mortality and the total burden of disease attributable to illicit drug use in some regions will, by necessity, be speculative.

Whilst this is true, there are also environmental, cultural, and behavioural factors that vary between countries, and will affect estimates made for those countries (Degenhardt et al., 2004a). One major factor that will affect mortality rates among illicit drug using populations is the provision of drug-dependence treatment. Enrolment in drug treatment has been associated with substantially reduced drug use, as well as reduced risk of overdose and acquiring human immunodeficiency virus (HIV) (Darke et al., 2005f; Flynn et al., 2003; Gossop et al., 1999, 2000; Gronbladh et al., 1990; Stewart et al., 2002; Teesson et al., in press; Ward et al., 1998). The extent to which drug treatment is provided in a country, and is able to be accessed by dependent drug users, will thus impact substantially upon the rates of drug-related mortality amongst these populations. Provision and access to treatment will vary greatly, even between countries that are broadly similar, and mortality rates may thus vary widely.

Similarly, countries differ substantially in relation to blood-borne disease prevention programmes, such as the provision of sterile injecting equipment to injecting drug users (IDU). To the extent that such programmes reduce rates of blood-borne viral infections amongst illicit drug users, and subsequent death, there will be an impact upon mortality rates. As with treatment, differences in approaches to the containment of blood-borne infections may be substantial between otherwise similar countries, facing similar viral threats.

While estimating illicit drug-related death rates raises problems, estimating the extent to which these rates exceed population rates is also problematic. Standardised mortality ratios (SMRs), the ratio of observed to expected deaths, are typically derived from studies conducted amongst European and North American drug using cohorts. Caution must be exercised when extrapolating these mortality ratios to other settings, particularly third world countries, as there will be substantial differences in population death rates in a country such as the US compared to poor countries with limited medical resources. Whilst, for example, heroin users may die at a rate 20 times greater than that seen amongst the general US population, the excess mortality due to heroin use may be substantially *lower* in a third world nation, as overall population mortality is substantially *higher*.

Cohort studies provide a valuable means of estimating illicit drug user mortality rates, and are used in meta-analyses to determine these rates (e.g. Hulse et al., 1999). Two points must be borne in mind here. First, for logistical reasons, most cohorts have been initially recruited through treatment populations. Those entering drug treatment may thus not reflect death rates seen amongst the broader illicit drug using population. Second, the majority of studies have focussed on opioid users, and relatively few studies have examined rates across different drug classes.

Finally, there are specific problems that relate to causal attribution. As discussed above, unless a case of suicide is by means of a drug overdose, the causal role of illicit drug use in such a death may be overlooked. Disease also presents problems, as it is a dynamic factor in such deaths. The acquired immune deficiency syndrome (AIDS) pandemic amongst IDU from the 1980s onwards changed the nature and rates of death amongst IDU, as have the new anti-retroviral regimes that have prolonged life amongst those infected with HIV. Finally, trauma, which is discussed in detail in a later chapter, is difficult to quantify in official statistics. Illicit drug use, and injecting drug use in particular, is likely to involve increased risk of death through injury or violence. It is unlikely that such deaths would be classified as drug-related in any official statistics. Rates of death through trauma are thus likely to be underestimated.

The above all indicate that a number of caveats must be borne in mind when estimating death rates amongst illicit drug users. In all likelihood, these estimates will be conservative. Despite these caveats, however, a large amount of data exists that can be considered. As will be seen, despite the above caveats, these studies show a large degree of consistency. All sources indicate high mortality rates amongst illicit drug using populations and, further, that these rates are greatly in excess of those of the general population. Given that, as will be seen in the ensuing chapters, there is wide and continuing exposure among illicit drug users to a range of mortality risk factors at rates far beyond those seen in the general population, these findings make causal sense. Whilst the specifics of drug-related deaths may be debated, and appropriate caveats borne in mind, the overall patterns and trends of such deaths are consistent and indicate a major clinical and social problem.

3.3   Mortality amongst illicit drug users

The most comprehensive attempt to quantify the global burden of disease, and more specifically of mortality, attributable to substance use and dependence was recently published by the World Health Organization (Ezzati et al., 2004).

Table 3.1. Deaths and Disability Adjusted Life Years (DALYs) attributed to illicit drug use in 2000, with comparisons to alcohol and tobacco

Region	Males (% of cases)	Females (% of cases)	All (% of cases)
Africa	23,828 (87.2)	3,504 (12.8)	27,332 (100)
Asia/Pacific	50,487 (83.6)	9,882 (16.4)	60,369 (100)
Europe	21,875 (66.4)	11,081 (35.6)	32,956 (100)
Middle East	12,797 (83.0)	2,626 (17.0)	15,423 (100)
North America	22,599 (56.0)	17,757 (44.0)	40,356 (100)
South/ Central America	13,424 (64.1)	7,523 (35.9)	20,947 (100)
Total illicit drug deaths[*]	145,010 (73.5)	52,373 (26.5)	197,383 (100)
DALYs	5,402,000	1,477,000	6,879,000
Alcohol[+] total deaths	1,638,000 (91)	166,000 (9)	1,804,000 (100)
DALYs	761,562,000	693,911,000	1,455,473,000
Tobacco[#] total deaths	3,840,000 (80)	1,000,000 (20)	4,830,000 (100)
DALYs	48,177,000	10,904,000	59,081,000

[*]Degenhardt et al. (2004a); [+]Rehm et al. (2004); [#]Ezzati, M. & Lopez, A. (2004).

Estimates were made of the mortality attributable to substance dependence in the year 2000, based upon a mixture of direct (e.g. specific cause of death figures, such as overdose) and indirect estimates (e.g. extrapolation of mortality rates form large cohort studies). On the basis of these analyses, it was estimated that 197,383 deaths that were attributable to illicit drug use occurred in 2000 alone (Table 3.1) (Degenhardt et al., 2004a). As would be expected, given the difficulties involved in making such estimates, there was a wide confidence interval around this estimate, with an upper estimate of 322,456 cases. As can be seen, and consistent with the rise in illicit drug use seen around the world (United Nations Office for Drug Control, 2005), illicit drug use deaths were not restricted to any one world region.

The same study also estimated the Disability Adjusted Life Years (DALYs) due to illicit drug use mortality. DALYs are defined as the sum of years of potential life lost due to premature mortality, and the years of productive life lost due to disability. They are thus a combination measure of lost life and disability. In 2000, it was estimated that over 6.87 million DALYs were attributable to illicit drug use, which represents 0.8% of all global DALYs for that year (Degenhardt et al., 2004a).

By way of comparison, Table 3.1 also presents mortality estimates for both alcohol (Rehm et al. 2004) and tobacco (Ezzati & Lopez, 2004). As would be expected, given the far more extensive use of these substances, the estimated mortality is substantially higher than for illicit drugs. In 2000, it was estimated that there were 1.8 million deaths attributable to alcohol and 4.8 million for tobacco. These licit substances thus clearly cause more deaths per year than do illicit drugs. However, despite the illicit nature of the drugs in question, and substantially lower prevalence of use, the estimated number of illicit drug deaths in 2000 was 11% of those attributed to alcohol.

Mortality rates of large-scale cohorts of illicit drug users are presented in Table 3.2. As can be seen, in the majority of studies the mortality rate exceeds 15 per thousand person years. How this compares to the general population is demonstrated by the SMRs pertaining to these studies. In all of these studies, mortality rates were far in excess of those seen amongst the general population of the countries in which they were conducted. In fact, in the majority of these studies the excess mortality was more than 10 times that of non-drug users matched for age and gender.

3.4 Factors associated with illicit drug-related mortality

3.4.1 Drug class

The nature and extent of risks associated with illicit drug use will clearly vary according to the type of substance used. Perhaps the major risk associated with opioid use is overdose, discussed in detail in Chapter 5, which constitutes a substantial proportion of opioid-related deaths. Overdose is also a risk for stimulant use, although the mechanisms differ from those of opioids, and there does not appear to be the clear dose response seen in opioids (cf. Chapter 4). Injectors of any drug will be at risk of infection with blood-borne viruses, such as HIV or hepatitis C, if they engage in the sharing of injecting equipment (Karch, 2002).

Deaths due to other drug classes are less well-documented than those seen amongst opioid and stimulant users. Whilst not large in number, deaths due to methylenedioxymethamphetamine (MDMA) have been documented, and have been related to cardiac arrhythmia, hyperthermic collapse, dehydration, or excessive water consumption (Karch, 2002; Schifano, 2004). Cannabis, the most widely used illicit drug, has no risk of overdose or infection through the sharing of injecting equipment. Cannabis-related mortality is primarily due to the long-term effects of route of administration on the respiratory system or traumatic motor vehicle accidents (Kalant et al., 1999; Kelly et al., 2004).

Table 3.2. All cause mortality rates amongst illicit drug user cohorts

Study	Country/Period	Sample	Drug	Standardized mortality ratio	Crude mortality rate (per 1000 person years)
Bargagli et al. (2001)	Italy 1980–1997	Treatment	Heroin	17.3; Male 15.4, Female 37.8	21.5
Bartu et al. (2004)	Australia 1985–1998	Hospital/psychiatric admissions	Opioids, amphetamine	–	1.8
Benson & Holmberg (1984)	Sweden 1968–1978	Conscripts, rehabilitation and psychiatric patients, welfare recipients	Cannabis, solvents, last stage of delirium (LSD), stimulants	26.0	4.5
Bewley et al. (1968)	UK 1947–1966	Notified addicts	Heroin	28.0	27.0
Brugal et al. (2005)	Spain 1992–1999	Treatment	Heroin	–	0.4
Bucknall & Robertson (1986)	UK 1981–1985	General Practitioner attendees	Heroin	11.6	9.7
Caplehorn et al. (1996)	Australia 1979–1991	Treatment	Heroin	–	12.1
Cherubin et al. (1972)	US 1964–1968	Notified addicts	Heroin	–	6.4–12.8
Concool et al. (1979)	US 1969–1976	Treatment	Heroin	1.5	5.6
Cotrell et al. (1985)	UK 1971–1982	Notified addicts	Heroin	–	18.6
Davoli et al. (1997)	Italy 1980–1992	Treatment	IDU	Male 21.2, Female 38.5	24.5
Dukes et al. (1992)	New Zealand 1971–1989	Treatment	Opioids	2.4; Male 1.8, Female 4.7	7.4
Engstrom et al. (1991)	Sweden 1973–1984	Drug-related hospitalisation	Amphetamine, cocaine, heroin	5.3; Male 5.8, Female 4.6	23.0
Eskild et al. (1993)	Norway 1985–1991	HIV test centre	IDU	31.0; Male 25.0, Female 58.0	23.5
Friedman et al. (1996)	US 1984–1992	Welfare recipients	Drugs and alcohol	5.2	28.4

(Contd.)

Table 3.2. (*Contd.*)

Study	Country/Period	Sample	Drug	Standardized mortality ratio	Crude mortality rate (per 1000 person years)
Frischer et al. (1997)	UK 1982–1994	Treatment	IDU	22.0; Male 16.1, Female 37.7	20.8
Fugelstad et al. (1995)	Sweden 1986–1990	HIV + drug addicts	Heroin	–	38.5
Fugelstad et al. (1997)	Sweden 1981–1992	Drug-related hospitalisation	Heroin, amphetamine	–	16.3
Galli & Musicco (1994)	Italy 1980–1991	Treatment	IDU	20.5; Male 19.5, Female 54.2	25.2
Ghodse et al. (1998)	UK 1967–1993	Notified "Drug addicts"	Opioids	7–13; Male 2.9–16.9, Female 5.0–21.0	7.7
Goedert et al. (1995)	Italy 1980–1990	Treatment	Heroin	18.0	15.7
Goldstein & Herrera (1995)	US 1979–1993	Treatment	Heroin	Male 4.0, Female 11.1	15.6
Gossop et al. (2002b)	UK 1995–1999	Treatment	Heroin, amphetamine	6.0	–
Gronbladh et al. (1990)	Sweden 1967–1988	Treatment, untreated	Heroin	63.1 (street), 8.4 (methadone)	29.2
Haarstrup & Jepson (1988)	Denmark 1973–1984	Treatment	Opioids	–	26.3
Hser et al. (1993)	US 1962–1986	Treatment	Narcotics	–	12.3
Joe et al. (1982)	US 1969–1979	Treatment	Opioids	1.7; Male 1.7, Female 1.8	15.2
Joe & Simpson (1987)	US 1978–1984	Treatment	Opioids	6.9	15.6
Langendam et al. (2001)	Holland, 1985–1996	Treatment/community	Heroin, cocaine	–	30.2
McAnulty et al. (1995)	US 1989–1991	Not in treatment	IDU	8.3	10.5
Musto & Ramos (1981)	US 1918–1973	Treatment	Morphine	–	8.4

Study	Country/Period	Setting	Drug	Rate detail	Mortality
Oppenheimer et al. (1994)	UK 1969–1991	Treatment	Heroin	11.9; Male 11.2 Female 13.9	15.3
Orti et al. (1996)	Spain 1985–1991	Treatment, Hospital	Opioids	–	30.1
Oyefesso et al. (1999b)	UK 1974–1993	Notified teenage addicts	Opioids	12.3; Male 10.7, Female 21.2	4.7
Perucci et al. (1991)	Italy 1980–1988	Treatment	Opioids	10.1; Male 9.3, Female 18.1	7.1
Quaglio et al. (2001)	Italy 1985–1998	Treatment	IDU	12.9; Male 8.9, Female 21.7	–
Rehm et al. (2005)	Switzerland 1994–2000	Treatment	Heroin	9.7; Male 8.4, Female 17.2	10.6
Rossow (1994)	Norway 1968–1992	Treatment	"Addicts"	–	24.0
Sanchez-Carbonell & Seus (2000)	Spain 1985–1995	Treatment	Heroin	28.5	34.0
Tunving (1988)	Sweden 1970–1984	Treatment	Opioids, amphetamine	5.4 (opiates) 2.5 (amphetamine)	11.8
Vaillant (1973)	US 1952–1970	Treatment, males	Narcotics	–	11.5
Van Ameijden et al. (1999a)	Holland 1985–1995	Treatment and community agencies	IDU	–	17.5
Van Haarstrecht et al. (1996)	Holland 1985–1993	Treatment, STD patients	IDU	–	25.9
Vlahov et al. (2004)	US 1988–2000	New onset IDU	IDU	3.1–8.1	32.6
Wahren et al. (1997)	Sweden 1970–1974	Hospitalised for drug dependence	Stimulants, opioids	6.9; Male 7.6, Female 5.4	15.9
Watterson et al. (1975)	US 1970–1974	Treatment	Opioids	–	13.0
Wille (1981)	UK 1969–1979	Treatment	Heroin	–	14.8
Zaccarelli et al. (1994)	Italy 1985–1991	Treatment	IDU	Male HIV + 30.3, HIV – 11.1 Female HIV + 19.4, HIV – 4.9	23.0
Zanis & Woody (1998)	US 1993–1994	Methadone	Heroin	–	25.6

In addition to the innate risks associated with a drug, the pattern of drug use in a particular country will greatly affect the distribution of drug-related death. In Europe, opioids are by far the principal cause of drug-related death (European Monitoring Centre for Drugs and Drug Addiction, 2004). By contrast, in the US opiates and cocaine figure prominently in deaths, most particularly in combination (Coffin et al., 2003; Department of Health and Human Services, 2005). In all of these regions, relatively small proportions of cases are attributed to amphetamine, MDMA, or cannabis.

When examining the rates of death due to different drugs, it must be borne in mind that polydrug use, of both licit and illicit substances, is the norm amongst illicit drug users (e.g. Darke & Hall, 1995; Darke & Ross, 1997; Dinwiddie et al., 1996; Gossop et al., 2002a; Hubbard et al., 1997; Klee et al., 1990; Ross & Darke, 2000). This makes attribution to a particular drug difficult in many cases. This is illustrated by the strong association between heroin and cocaine seen in the US and elsewhere (Coffin et al., 2003; Darke et al., 2005a). Also, the caveats regarding hidden populations must be borne in mind. National statistics on illicit drug deaths will be biased towards clear overdoses, so may not reflect the overall mortality associated with a particular drug.

Few cohort studies have directly compared mortality rates across drug classes, a possible reflection of the predominance of opiate users in such cohorts. The few that have, however, consistently report significantly higher death rates amongst primary opiate users, but also report elevated death rates for stimulant users (Bartu et al., 2004; Engstrom et al., 1991; Fugelstad et al., 1997; Tunving, 1988; Wahren et al., 1997). Bartu et al. (2004) reported that opiate users were 1.4 times more likely to die than amphetamine users in their cohort, and were 2.4 times more likely to die from overdose. Fugelstad et al. (1997) also reported a substantially higher mortality rate (3.2 times) amongst opiate users when compared to amphetamine users. Many of the deaths amongst primary amphetamine users in this study were, in fact, due to heroin overdose, a good illustration of the problems polydrug use presents for causal attribution. Higher SMRs amongst opiate compared to stimulant users were reported by Engstrom et al. (1991) (18 versus 9), Tunving (1988) (5 versus 2.5), and Wahren et al. (1997) (22 versus 10). Overall, the data indicate that opiate use carries the highest risk of death, and overdose is the obvious candidate to explain this elevated risk (Bartu et al., 2004; Engstrom et al., 1991; Fugelstad et al., 1997; Tunving, 1988; Wahren et al., 1997).

More widespread polydrug use appears to increase the risk of death amongst illicit drug users (Gossop et al., 2002a; Van Ameijden et al., 1999a; van Haarstrecht et al., 1996). In particular, heavy alcohol use (Cooncool et al., 1979; Friedman et al., 1996; Gossop et al., 2002a; Hser et al., 1998, 2001; Joe et al.,

1982; Musto & Ramos, 1981; van Ameijdan et al., 1999a; van Haarstrecht et al., 1996) and benzodiazepine use (Caplehorn, 1996; Gossop et al., 2002a; van Ameijdan et al., 1999a; van Haarstrecht et al., 1996) appear to substantially increase mortality rates. A partial explanation for these findings is that both alcohol and benzodiazepines are central nervous system (CNS) depressants, and increase the risk of overdose when used in conjunction with opioids. Concomitant alcohol use also increases the toxicity of cocaine, and is strongly associated with cocaine toxicity deaths (Coffin et al., 2003; Darke et al., 2005a; Karch, 2002). Heavy alcohol use is also associated with liver disease, while both alcohol and benzodiazepine dependence increase the risk of suicide (Harris & Barraclough, 1997). There is also a strong relationship between these drugs and death due to trauma (Gill, 2001; Greenberg et al., 1999; Kelly et al., 2004). Given all this, when these licit substances are used in combination with illicit drugs, it is not surprising that the risk of death increases. The relationship between polydrug use and mortality is crucial, and is discussed further throughout this book.

3.4.2 Gender

Consistent with the epidemiology of illicit drug use (Chapter 2), the majority of deaths worldwide attributable to illicit drug use occur amongst males (Table 3.1). These estimates indicate that males constitute approximately three quarters of deaths, and of DALYs. Males have also dominated deaths in the major cohort studies (Table 3.3), ranging to 87% of cases (Gossop et al., 2002b).

Whilst males constitute the bulk of fatal cases, the SMRs associated with *female* mortality are generally greater than those of males (Table 3.2). The discrepancy between male and female SMRs has been consistently reported in studies from different countries, and is quite pronounced in many studies, for example, 15.4 versus 37.8 (Bargagli et al., 2001), 21.2 versus 38.5 (Davoli et al., 1997), 4.0 versus 11.1 (Goldstein & Herrera, 1995), 8.4 versus 17.2 (Rehm et al., 2005). What this means is that female illicit drug users are substantially more likely to die than non-drug using females, than are males when compared to non-drug using males. Thus, in the Bargagli et al. (2001) study, female drug users were 37 times more likely to die than non-drug using females, while males in the cohort were 15 times more likely to die than non-drug using males.

The fact that males represent the majority of fatalities is expected, as they constitute the majority of illicit drug users. How, then, do we interpret the reverse situation in the case of SMRs? There are two possibilities. First, the female illicit drug users are more risky than their male counterparts. The fact that females are substantially less likely to use illicit drugs than males may mean that those

Table 3.3. Demographic characteristics of illicit drug-related deaths in major cohort studies

Study	Country/Period	Drug	Mean age at death	Gender (% male)
Bargagli et al. (2001)	Italy 1980–1997	Heroin	32.9	81
Bartu et al. (2004)	Australia 1985–1998	Opioids, amphetamine	34.6	66
Benson & Holmberg (1984)	Sweden 1968–1978	Cannabis, solvents, LSD, stimulants	–	84
Brugal et al. (2005)	Spain 1992–1999	Heroin	39.0	77
Bucknall & Robertson (1986)	UK 1981–1985	Heroin	Male 28.3 Female 22.0	86
Cherubin et al. (1972)	US 1964–1968	Heroin	28.3	85
Cooncool et al. (1979)	US 1969–1976	Heroin	35.1	–
Cottrell et al. (1985)	UK 1971–1982	Heroin	29.9	–
Davoli et al. (1997)	Italy 1980–1992	IDU	–	83
Dukes et al. (1992)	New Zealand 1971–1989	Opioids	32.3	69
Engstrom et al. (1991)	Sweden 1973–1984	Amphetamine, cocaine, heroin	–	66
Eskild et al. (1993)	Norway 1985–1991	IDU	–	65
Friedman et al. (1996)	US 1984–1992	Drugs and alcohol	–	79
Frischer et al. (1997)	UK 1982–1994	IDU	26.3	66
Fugelstad et al. (1997)	Sweden 1981–1992	Heroin, amphetamine	–	75

Galli & Musicco (1994)	Italy 1980–1991	IDU	–	82
Ghodse et al. (1998)	UK 1967–1993	Opioids	30.6	78
Gossop et al. (2002b)	UK 1995–1999	Heroin, amphetamine	30.6	87
Gronbladh et al. (1990)	Sweden 1967–1988	Heroin	–	80
Hser et al. (1993)	US 1962–1986	Narcotics	40.2	–
McAnulty et al. (1995)	US 1989–1991	IDU	–	73
Musto & Ramos (1981)	US 1918–1973	Morphine	55.9	–
Oppenheimer et al. (1994)	UK 1969–1991	Heroin	–	70
Orti et al. (1996)	Spain 1985–1991	Opioids	–	75
Oyefesso et al. (1999a)	UK 1974–1993	Opioids	23.0	76
Perucci et al. (1991)	Italy 1980–1988	Opioids	–	84
Quaglio et al. (2001)	Italy 1985–1998	IDU	31.3	84
Rossow (1994)	Norway 1968–1992	"Addicts"	–	81
Sanchez-Carbonell & Seus (2000)	Spain 1985–1995	Heroin	31.0	76
Tunving (1988)	Sweden 1970–1984	Opioids, amphetamine	27.6	84
Van Haarstrecht et al. (1996)	Holland 1985–1993	IDU	–	68
Wahren et al. (1997)	Sweden	Stimulants, opioids	–	75
Wille (1981)	UK 1969–1979	Heroin	30.8	74
Zaccarelli et al. (1994)	Italy 1985–1991	IDU	–	79

who do so are a self-selected, and riskier population than the more commonly seen male drug user. Several factors, however, contradict this possibility. The prevalence of the psychiatric diagnoses that most directly measure impulsivity, risk, and deviance (Antisocial Personality Disorder (ASPD) and Borderline Personality Disorder (BPD)) in many studies are no higher amongst female drug users than amongst males (Darke et al., 1998, 2005d; Gill et al., 1992; Luthar et al., 1996). If females were comparatively more "deviant" than males, we would most certainly expect to see higher rates of these disorders.

More importantly, when gender-specific mortality rates have been reported, or the gender proportions of deaths compared to baseline, there is no observable difference between male and female death rates (Bargagli et al., 2001; Bartu et al., 2004; Caplehorn 1996; Frischer et al., 1997; Fugelstad et al., 1997; Galli & Mustico, 1994; Goldstein & Herrara, 1995; Gossop et al., 2002a; Gronbladh et al., 1990; McAnulty et al., 1995; Oppenheimer et al., 1994; Orti et al., 1996; Oyefesso et al., 1999a; Perucci et al., 1991; Rossow, 1994; Sanchez-Carbonell & Seus, 2000; Tunving 1988; Van Haarstrecht et al., 1996; Wahren et al., 1997; Watterson et al., 1975; Wille, 1981; Zaccarelli et al., 1994). If anything, these studies indicate slightly *higher* rates amongst males. Thus, females *within* drug using cohorts appear no more likely to die than male members of the cohort.

The more likely explanation for higher female SMRs is the lower base population mortality rates seen amongst females. If the mortality rates of male and female illicit drug users are similar, then the SMRs of females drug users will be far greater compared to other females, than for male drug users compared to other males. While the chances of death may be similar for both male and female drugs users, the excess risk faced by females compared to their non-drug using female peers is substantially greater than that seen among males.

3.4.3   Age

In overall population terms, most deaths due to illicit drug use occur among the young. As can be seen from Table 3.3, the mean age at death in cohort studies has been generally in the vicinity of 30 years. An average age of death around 30 is consistent with studies of illicit drug-related fatalities (e.g. Darke & Zador, 1996; Karch et al., 1999; Schifano, 2004), and with estimates indicating that the highest proportion of deaths occur in the 25–34 and 25–44 years age brackets (Degenhardt et al., 2004a). The fact that these deaths occur amongst a relatively young age group is reflected in the large number of DALYs attributable to illicit drugs (Table 3.1).

Whilst in overall population terms these deaths occur among the young, in the context of drug using careers these are older, experienced drug users. As discussed previously, illicit drug use typically commences in the early- to mid-teenage years (Chen & Kandel, 1995; Degenhardt et al., 2000; Kandel et al., 1992). These deaths thus typically occur amongst a group that has been using illicit drugs for a decade or more. It is not the new, inexperienced user who appears to be most at risk, despite the pervasiveness of this view in media coverage which emphasises cases of very young illicit drug-related deaths. The bulk of cases occur amongst older drug users. Consistent with these findings, cohort studies of illicit drug users have repeatedly reported older age as an independent predictor of death during follow-up (Bartu et al., 2004; Brugal et al., 2005; Cooncool et al., 1979; Davoli et al., 1997; Dukes et al., 1992; Eskild et al., 1993; Friedman et al., 1996; Frischer et al., 1997; Gossop et al., 2002a; Goedert et al., 1995; Hser et al., 2001; Joe & Simpson, 1987; Joe et al., 1982; McAnulty et al., 1995; Oppenheimer et al., 1994; Quaglio et al., 2001; Watterson et al., 1975; Wahren et al., 1997; Zacarelli et al., 1994).

Why are older illicit drug users most at risk? When considering this we must remember that, whilst older, these deaths are not due to advanced age, which would be unremarkable. It is the period between the teenage years and the early 30s that is of most interest here. To comprehensively answer why it is older users who are most at risk, we must examine the causes of death, as will be done in detail in later chapters. Several possible factors emerge. First, there is the possibility of disease progression, particularly due to HIV or hepatitis C (Chapter 5). Older users may be sicker, and die due to illness. Second, the finding may relate to the cumulative risk associated with illicit drug use. In particular, the cumulative risk of overdose may be such that the risk of death is substantially higher at 30 than at 18. This finding may also represent some aspect of the natural history of illicit drug use, such as increased risk of overdose in later career stages (cf. Chapter 4). Of course, these potential explanations are not mutually exclusive. A person with hepatitis C may well be at greater risk of an overdose due to liver damage as the disease progresses. Whatever the case, when considering means by which to reduce illicit drug-related mortality, it must be borne in mind that it is the longer-term drug user who presents the highest risk, and is a major target for intervention.

3.4.4   *Length of drug use career*

A risk factor that is related to, but not identical with, age is the length of drug use career. Effectively this is the period between current age and the age of initiation

of drug use. As discussed in Chapter 1, illicit drug use careers are complex, and
may include many cyclical periods of drug use, treatment, and abstinence
(Darke et al., 2005c; Flynn et al., 2003; Hser et al., 2001). Longer length of career
has, however, repeatedly been related to a higher risk of mortality (Brugal
et al., 2005; Caplehorn et al., 1996; Cooncool et al., 1979; Eskild et al., 1993;
Hser et al., 2001; McAnulty et al., 1995; Orti et al., 1996; Quaglio et al., 2001;
van Haarstrecht et al., 1996; Vlahov et al., 2004). As was seen with age, it is not
new users who are at the greatest risk of mortality. More so than age, length of
drug use career is probably a proxy for cumulative risk exposure from factors
such as overdose, viral infection, and trauma. A longer length of career may
also reflect increased drug dependence and more problematic use, with consequent increased risk of death.

The findings from cohort studies on mortality risk relating to both age and
length of use career indicate that it is the older, experienced user who is at greatest risk. It is important to note, however, that in recent years the age of initiation
to both licit and illicit drug use has declined in many countries (Degenhardt
et al., 2000). Such a trend has two implications. First, the age of death of drug
users may begin to decline, as exposure to risks such as overdose and disease
commences earlier. Second, earlier age of onset of drug use has been associated
with higher levels of dependence and with more serious drug-related problems
(Fergusson & Horwood, 1997; Grant & Dawson, 1998; Mills et al., 2004). After
a decade of heroin use, for example, a heroin user who commenced use at age
15 will generally have more serious drug-dependency problems than one who
commenced at 20. The consequences of earlier onset of drug use would, in all
probability, exacerbate any trend towards earlier death amongst these populations. Indeed, such a trend has already been noted. In Australia, between the
early 1970s and late 1990s, the age of death declined for each succeeding birth
cohort (Hall et al., 1999a).

3.4.5 Drug-dependence treatment

One factor that appears to reduce mortality is treatment for drug dependence.
Cohort studies have consistently found that retention in drug-treatment programmes substantially reduces mortality risk (Bartu et al., 2004; Brugal et al.,
2005; Caplehorn et al., 1996; Davoli et al., 1993; Esteban et al., 2003; Fugelstad
et al., 1995, 1997; Gronbladh et al., 1990; Quaglio et al., 2001; Segest et al.,
1990; Watterson et al., 1975; Zanis & Woody, 1998). The extent of this reduction in mortality risk was illustrated dramatically by Gronbladh et al. (1990)
in relation to methadone maintenance. Not in treatment "street" users had an

elevated rate of death 63 times that of the general population, compared to an 8-fold risk amongst those enrolled in treatment. Similarly, Zanis & Woody (1998) reported that 8% of patients discharged from methadone maintenance died over 12 months, compared to only 1% of those enrolled in treatment. Whilst treatment clearly cannot reduce the excess risk of death seen amongst illicit drug users to zero, cohort studies indicate that it does substantially reduce this risk. It should not, however, be assumed that any or all drug treatment reduces mortality risk. Rather, in the studies cited above it is prolonged, stable treatment that is most effective in reducing mortality risk. Indeed, as will be discussed in Chapter 4, there are specific situations in which mortality risk may actually *increase* (e.g. the induction phase of methadone, cessation of naltrexone maintenance). Despite these specific situations, the overall effect of treatment upon mortality is positive.

Why does stable drug treatment have such an impact upon mortality? This issue will be more fully explored in Chapter 8. Briefly, however, treatment outcome studies have repeatedly demonstrated that enrolment in the major treatment modalities is associated with large reductions in drug use (e.g. Darke et al., 2005c; Flynn et al., 2003; Gossop et al., 1999; Hubbard et al., 1997; Teesson et al., 2006). As well as substantial reductions in drug use, these studies also document reductions in crime, sharing of injecting equipment, psychopathology, as well as improvements in physical health. Better treatment outcomes have been associated with longer retention times and stability of treatment (Darke et al., 2005c; Flynn et al., 2003; Gossop et al., 1999; Hubbard et al., 1997; Simpson et al., 1997).

The reduction in mortality risk factors associated with drug treatment (Table 3.4) is of particular relevance. One major factor that treatment appears to impact upon is overdose. As will be discussed in Chapter 4, overdose represents a major cause of death amongst drug users, particularly opioid and cocaine users. Treatment has been demonstrated to reduce the risk of non-fatal overdose (Darke et al., 2005f; Stewart et al., 2002) and fatal overdose cases are rarely in drug treatment (Darke & Zador, 1996; Darke et al., 2005a; Davidson et al., 2003). This reduction in overdose risk is probably due to reduced rates of drug use and, in the case of opioid agonist therapies, a correspondingly high tolerance to opioids. Treatment has also been demonstrated to be protective against HIV infection, a consequence of the substantially reduced rates of sharing of injecting equipment associated with treatment (Ward et al., 1998). Two positive consequences of treatment for drug use then, are reductions in risk of death by overdose and disease. A recent study of the impact of drug treatment on suicide risk, however, indicated that treatment did not significantly reduce this risk

Table 3.4. Factors associated with illicit drug-related mortality

Risk factor	Comment
Drug class	Highest risk for opiates
Gender	Males comprise the majority of fatalities. SMRs of females higher than males.
Age	Higher risk for older drug users, with average age of death around 30 years.
Length of use career	Longer drug use careers associated with greater risk.
Treatment	Enrolment in drug treatment associated with substantially lower risk of death.
HIV infection	Higher mortality rates amongst HIV positive drug users.
Psychosocial functioning	Poorer psychosocial functioning associated with increased risk of death.

(Darke et al., 2005e) (cf. Chapter 6). The effects of treatment upon trauma risk have not been quantified to date.

3.4.6 Disease

Illicit drug use is associated with increased risk for a range of diseases (Cherubin & Sapira, 1993; Karch, 2002). Most prominent amongst these is infection with HIV, hepatitis B and hepatitis C, transmitted through injecting with used injecting equipment and/or unprotected sexual activity. There are also specific pathologies related to the use of individual drugs. Cocaine and, to a lesser extent, amphetamine are cardiotoxic, and strongly associated with accelerated atherosclerosis, cerebrovascular accident, cardiomegaly, and cardiac infarction (Karch, 2002). There are also significant health effects of cannabis that relate to smoking as a route of administration (Kalant et al., 1999).

The impact of disease upon illicit drug user mortality is substantial (cf. Chapter 5), as the proportion of deaths attributable to disease illustrates, for example, Bargagli et al. (2001) (30%), Maxwell et al., (2005) (62%), Hser et al. (2001) (40%), Goedert et al. (1995) (73%). Since the advent of the HIV pandemic a large proportion, and in many studies the majority of disease-related deaths (e.g. Bargagli et al., 2001; Brugal et al., 2005; Davoli et al., 1997; Friedman et al., 1996; Vlahov et al., 2004), have been attributable to the consequences of HIV infection (Chapter 5).

The range of cohort studies that have examined baseline health status and risk of mortality is not extensive, and has overwhelmingly focused on baseline

HIV serostatus. Not surprisingly, given the risk to life it represents, positive HIV status is associated with significantly higher mortality rates (Eskild et al., 1993; Esteban et al., 2003; Friedman et al., 1996; Frischer et al., 1993, 1997; Fugelstad et al., 1997; Galli & Musicco, 1994; Goedert et al., 1995; Langendam et al., 2001; Orti et al., 1996; Quaglio et al., 2001; van Ameijdan et al., 1999a; van Haarstrecht et al., 1996; Vlahov et al., 2004; Zacarelli et al., 1994). For example, Vlahov et al. (2004) reported that mortality rates among HIV-positive cohort members were 7.3 times those of HIV negative cohort members. Similarly high excess mortality ratios amongst the HIV positive have also been consistently reported in other studies (e.g. Eskild et al., 1993; Esteban et al., 2003; Fugelstad et al., 1997). While the mortality rates of HIV negative drug users exceed those of the general population, rates among the HIV positive are elevated further. It is important to note that this excess mortality is not solely related to AIDS. Whilst not always noted, higher death rates amongst the HIV positives from causes other than AIDS have been reported by Eskild et al. (1993), Goedert et al. (1995), Quaglio et al. (2001), and Zacarelli et al. (1994).

On a broader level, both Hser et al. (1994, 2001) reported that physical disability amongst opiate users that was sufficient to interfere with holding a job increased the risk of mortality by 3.6 and 2.7 times respectively. Poorer global physical health has also been associated with an increased risk of death (Gossop et al., 2002a; Langendam et al., 2001). Both Langedam et al. (2001) and Van Haarstrecht et al. (1996) reported that being clinically underweight, a probable marker for poor health, was an independent predictor of mortality, even after controlling for HIV status.

3.4.7 *Psychosocial functioning*

The demographic characteristics of drug-related deaths typically reflect lower psychosocial functioning (Bartu et al., 2004; Darke & Zador, 1996; Darke & Ross, 2002; Davoli et al., 1993). Opioid overdose deaths predominantly occur among long-term, dependent, socially isolated heroin users with prison histories, who are typically unemployed as is also the case with cocaine (cf. Chapter 4). Suicide is strongly associated with poorer psychosocial functioning, social isolation, and psychological distress, both amongst the general population and amongst drug users in particular (cf. Chapter 6). Overall, the profile of drug user deaths suggests low levels of psychosocial functioning.

Few cohort studies have specifically related psychosocial functioning to mortality, reflecting an absence of good data on these variables. Those studies that have examined these factors, however, are consistent with the profile of deaths due to illicit drugs derived form retrospective studies (Bartu et al., 2004; Davoli et al., 1993; Gossop et al., 2002a; Harlow, 1990; Haarstrup & Jepson, 1988; Kjelsberg et al., 1995; Langendam et al., 2001; Musto & Ramos, 1981; Segest et al., 1990; van Haarstrecht et al., 1996; Zanis & Woody, 1998). Even within a population that has high levels of social disadvantage and psychopathology, psychosocial dysfunction still predicts mortality. Periods of homelessness are common amongst dependent illicit drug users, and have been associated with increased risk of premature mortality (Darke & Ross, 2001; Gossop et al., 2002a; Langendam et al., 2001). This may partially reflect the fact that homelessness is a risk factor for suicide, both amongst the general population, and amongst illicit drug users in particular (Darke et al., 2001). Street injecting, a concomitant of homelessness amongst IDU, has also been associated with higher overdose risk and poorer vascular health (Darke et al., 2001; Klee & Morris, 1995). Homelessness also exposes an individual to greater risk of trauma and disease.

Unemployment and lower income levels have been specifically related to risk of mortality (Harlow, 1990; Musto & Ramos, 1981). It will also be recalled that disability sufficient to interfere with holding employment increases mortality risk (Hser et al., 1998, 2001). A lower level of education, a probable marker for lower income and/or unemployment, has also been associated with increased mortality risk (Davoli et al., 1993).

Poorer global psychosocial functioning has been specifically related to increased mortality risk (Haarstrup & Jepson, 1988), having unstable social groupings (Segest et al., 1990) and being single (Davoli et al., 1993; van Haarstrecht et al., 1996). Whilst the latter reflects the risks associated with lower levels of social support, it may also reflect the risk of fatal overdose when others are not available to intervene. This is clearly less likely when the drug user has a partner.

As mentioned earlier, illicit drug use is associated with high levels of psychopathology, particularly mood and anxiety disorders (Darke & Ross, 2001; Degenhardt et al., 2001; Dinwiddie et al., 1992; Teesson et al., 2005). Major depression, a common diagnosis amongst the dependent drug users who comprise the bulk of mortality cases, is a strong risk factor for attempted and completed suicide (Harris & Barraclough, 1997) and overdose (Best et al., 2000). Few cohort studies have measured psychopathology as a risk factor for mortality. Those that have, however, have reported an increased risk associated with psychiatric hospital admission (Bartu et al., 2004), major depression (Kjelsberg et al., 1995, Zanis & Woody, 1998), and anxiety (Gossop et al., 2002a).

Overall, dependent illicit drug use is associated with a poor psychosocial profile. Even within this population, however, a poorer psychosocial profile appears to further increase the risk of premature death.

3.5 Major causes of death amongst illicit drug users

It is apparent from the preceding sections that mortality rates amongst illicit drug users far exceed those seen amongst the general population. What then are the main causes of these elevated rates? These fall into four main areas: drug overdose, disease, suicide, and trauma. A brief overview of how these areas relate to drug users is presented below. Cause-specific death rates, epidemiology, toxicology, and risk factors for each of these areas will be fully explored in Chapters 4–7.

3.5.1 Drug overdose

Drug overdose is an area that, by definition, is specifically relevant to drug users. Overdose is clearly not going to be a cause of death amongst those who do not use such substances. In particular, overdose is a major cause of premature death among opioid users and cocaine users. Whilst less common, death due to the toxicity of amphetamine, or MDMA and other "party" drugs, does occur. Cannabis, whilst the most widely used illicit drug, is not a drug that causes overdose death, and does not figure in subsequent discussions of overdose. Drug overdose as a cause of death is explored fully in Chapter 4.

3.5.2 Disease

Unlike overdose, disease as a cause of death is relevant to both drug users and non-drug users alike. There are, however, specific disease risks associated with illicit drug use that occur at much lower levels amongst the general population. In particular, injecting drug use is strongly associated with the transmission of blood-borne viruses, such as HIV, HCV, and HBV. Disease as a cause of death is fully explored in Chapter 5.

3.5.3 Suicide

Suicide is a leading cause of death amongst illicit drug users, and occurs at rates far in excess of those of the general population (Chapter 6). This is not surprising, as amongst this group rates of psychopathology (and major depression in particular) far exceed those in the non-drug using population. In addition, illicit drug users (opioid and cocaine users in particular), typically exhibit high levels of other risk factors for suicide. Despite high rates of suicide, and high rates of predisposing risk factors, suicide as a cause of death amongst injecting illicit drug users is substantially under-explored. Suicide as a cause of death is discussed fully in Chapter 6.

3.5.4   *Trauma*

There are a number of lifestyle factors surrounding illicit drug use that suggest that trauma may play a significant part in illicit drug user deaths. These include violence surrounding the use and procurement of highly expensive illegal drugs, high levels of risk due to crime and sex work performed to support drug use, high rates of psychiatric diagnoses that predispose individuals to impulsivity and violence, and the specific psychotropic effects of psychostimulant drugs. In addition, there is also a strong association between illicit drug use, motor vehicle trauma, and other traumatic events. Trauma as a cause of death is explored in Chapter 7.

3.6   Summary of illicit drug mortality

Estimating mortality attributable to illicit drug use is problematic due to factors such as these being hidden populations, differences in the quality of national official statistics, national differences in the provision of drug intervention programmes, and the inherent limitations of cohort studies. Within these limitations, however, it was estimated that approximately 200,000 deaths occurred in 2000 alone that were attributable to illicit drug use, representing over 6 million DALYs. The mortality rate in the majority of cohort studies exceeds 15 per thousand person years, with rates typically more than 10 times those of non-drug users. The majority of illicit drug-related deaths occur in males, the average age of death is in the vicinity of 30 years, and the highest risk of death is associated with opioid use. Factors that predict premature mortality include: being older, longer illicit drug use career, not being enrolled in a drug treatment programme, poorer health, and poorer psychosocial functioning. The major causes of death amongst illicit drug users are drug overdose, disease, suicide, and trauma.

Key points: Summary of all cause illicit drug-related mortality

- It is estimated that there were 197,383 deaths worldwide attributable to illicit drug use in the year 2000 alone.
- These deaths were responsible for the total of 6,879,000 years of lost life and productive life in 2000.
- Approximately three quarters of cases are male, and the mean age at death is approximately 30 years old.
- Opioids are associated with the highest risk of death.
- Predictors of mortality include older age, longer illicit drug use careers, not being enrolled in drug treatment, poorer health, and poorer psychosocial functioning.
- The major causes of death amongst drug users are drug overdose, disease, suicide, and trauma.

4

Mortality and drug overdose

4.1 Introduction

The current chapter examines mortality attributable to drug overdose, the dynamics of which are still poorly understood. The two main drug classes implicated, and the ones upon which the most work has been conducted, are opioids and cocaine. Fatal overdoses from amphetamine toxicity, and from methylenedioxymethamphetamine (MDMA) and other so-called "party drugs", are less well documented. In any discussion of overdose mortality, it is also clearly important to examine the related issue of non-fatal overdose. Non-fatal overdose is a far more common occurrence than fatal overdose, and is associated with a range of serious sequelae.

4.2 Rates of overdose

Opioid overdose is a major cause of premature death among heroin users (European Monitoring Centre for Drugs and Drug Addiction, 2004; US Department of Health and Human Services, 2005), and there have been strong trends internationally for the rates of such deaths to have increased dramatically in recent decades (Coffin et al., 2003; Drucker, 1999; Hall et al., 2000; Hickman et al., 2003; Preti et al., 2002; Steentoft et al., 1996). By way of example, between 1985–1995 the percentage of all deaths in Britain attributed to opioid overdose increased from 0.02% to 0.12%, and in Australia from 0.2 to 0.5% (Hall et al., 2000). It is important to note that the observed increases in opioid-related death rates were not restricted to illicit opioids. Increases in the numbers of overdose deaths due to methadone and, more recently, buprenorphine, have also been observed (Hall et al., 2000; Hickman et al., 2003; Kintz, 2001).

Over the preceding two decades cocaine has also emerged to become a major cause of mortality (Coffin et al., 2003; European Monitoring Centre for Drugs and

Drug Addiction, 2004; Sanchez et al., 1995; Tardiff et al., 1996; US Department of Health and Human Services, 2005). This is particularly true of the US, where cocaine is implicated in the majority of drug overdose deaths (Coffin et al., 2003). Cocaine-related deaths have also increased substantially in Europe and Australia (Darke et al., 2005a; European Monitoring Centre for Drugs and Drug Addiction, 2004).

While opioids and cocaine dominate illicit drug-related overdose deaths (European Monitoring Centre for Drugs and Drug Addiction, 2004; US Department of Health and Human Services, 2005) significant numbers of hospital admissions and deaths attributable to amphetamine toxicity do occur, and appear to be increasing, reflecting the renewed popularity of amphetamines (Degenhardt et al., 2005g; European Monitoring Centre for Drugs and Drug Addiction, 2004; Karch, 2002; Karch et al., 1999; National Institute on Drug Abuse, 2003; US Department of Health and Humans Services, 2005).

Apart from opiates, cocaine and amphetamine, the other class of drugs of interest for this book are "party drugs". Of this diverse class, the major drug of interest is MDMA ("ecstasy"). To date, no cohort studies have been conducted amongst users of MDMA. Reflecting the rarity of fatal MDMA overdose (compared to opiates, cocaine, and amphetamine) few case series have been reported (Gill et al., 2002; Lora-Tamayo et al., 1997; Schifano et al., 2003a, b), with most available data being individual case reports (e.g. Duflou & Mark, 2000; Fineschi & Masti, 1995). It is important to note, however, that such deaths do occur, and appear to have increased in number in recent years (Gill et al., 2002; Gowing et al., 2002; Karch, 2002; Schifano et al., 2003a, b; Schifano, 2004). By way of illustration, in England and Wales the number of MDMA-related deaths increased from 12 in 1996 to 72 in 2002 (Schifano et al., 1993a). The use of other party drugs, such as gamma-hydroxybutyrate (GHB) or ketamine, is comparatively rare compared to MDMA (Copeland & Dillon, 2005; Degenhardt et al., 2003), as are deaths from these drugs (Gill & Stajic, 2000; Karch, 2002). The remainder of this chapter will focus on MDMA as the party drug of clinical relevance.

The impact of overdose as a cause of death amongst illicit drug using cohorts is illustrated in Table 4.1. The proportion of deaths attributable to overdose has ranged up to 86% of cases amongst coronial studies (Marx et al., 1994), and 80% amongst cohorts (Gronbladh et al., 1990). In the majority of studies, the crude overdose specific mortality rate exceeded 5 per thousand person years. These rates dramatically illustrate the fact that overdose is a major component of the substantial excess mortality seen amongst illicit drug users described in Chapter 3, and is a major clinical issue in its own right.

Table 4.1. Overdose as a cause of death amongst illicit drug users

Study	Country/Period	Sample	Drug	Crude mortality rate (per 1000 person years)	Proportion of deaths due to overdose (%)
Bargagli et al. (2001)	Italy 1980–1997	Treatment	Heroin	5.2	24
Bartu et al. (2004)	Australia 1985–1998	Hospital/psychiatric admissions	Opioids, amphetamine	0.7	40
Benson & Holmberg (1984)	Sweden 1968–1978	Conscripts, rehabilitation and psychiatric patients, welfare recipients	Cannabis, solvents, lysergic acid diethylamide (LSD), stimulants	0.5	23
Bentley & Busuttil (1996)	UK 1989–1994	Coronial cases	Opioids	n/a	70
Bewley et al. (1968)	UK 1947–1966	Notified addicts	Heroin	7.9	29
Brugal et al. (2005)	Spain 1992–1999	Treatment	Heroin	0.2	35
Bucknall & Robertson (1986)	UK 1981–1985	General Practitioner (GP) attendees	Heroin	5.5	57
Caplehorn et al. (1996)	Australia 1979–1991	Treatment	Heroin	6.6	55
Cherubin et al. (1972)	USA 1964–1968	Notified addicts	Heroin	–	78
Concool et al. (1979)	USA 1969–1976	Treatment	Heroin	0.7	13
Davoli et al. (1997)	Italy 1980–1992	Treatment	Injecting drug users (IDU)	5.8	33
Darke et al. (2005a)	Australia 1993–2002	Coronial cases	Cocaine	n/a	86
Dukes et al. (1992)	New Zealand 1971–1989	Treatment	Opioids	2.5	37

Study	Country/period	Sample	Drug		
Engstrom et al. (1991)	Sweden 1973–1984	Drug-related hospitalisation	Amphetamine, cocaine, heroin	1.6	51 (poisoning + injury)
Eskild et al. (1993)	Norway 1985–1991	HIV test centre	IDU	15.6	67
Friedman et al. (1996)	USA 1984–1992	Welfare recipients	Drugs and alcohol	2.0	7
Frischer et al. (1997)	UK 1982–1994	Treatment	IDU	13.3	64
Fugelstad et al. (1995)	Sweden 1986–1990	HIV + drug addicts	Heroin	22.9	59
Fugelstad et al. (1997)	Sweden 1981–1992	Drug-related hospitalisation	Heroin, amphetamine	8.2	50
Galli & Musicco (1994)	Italy 1980–1991	Treatment	Methadone	9.2	37
Gardner (1970)	UK 1965–1969	Coronial cases	Opioids	n/a	57
Ghodse et al. (1998)	UK 1967–1993	Notified "Drug addicts"	Opioids	3.8	68
Gill et al. (2002)	USA 1997–2000	Coronial	MDMA	n/a	68
Goedert et al. (1995)	Italy 1980–1990	Treatment	Heroin	3.0	23
Goldstein & Herrera (1995)	USA 1979–1993	Treatment	Heroin	5.3	34
Gossop et al. (2002b)	UK 1995–1999	Treatment	Heroin, amphetamine	–	68
Gronbladh et al. (1990)	Sweden 1967–1988	Treatment, untreated	Heroin	17.4	80
Haarstrep & Jepson (1988)	Denmark 1973–1984	Treatment	Opioids	13.7	69
Hser et al. (1993)	USA 1962–1986	Treatment	Narcotics	4.0	32
Hser et al. (2001)	USA 1962–1997	Treatment	Narcotics	6.4	43
Joe et al. (1982)	USA 1969–1979	Treatment	Opioids	5.9	44 ("drug-related")
Joe & Simpson (1987)	USA 1978–1984	Treatment	Opioids	7.5	48 ("drug-related")
Karch et al. (1999)	USA 1985–1997	Coronial	Amphetamine	n/a	61

(*contd.*)

Table 4.1. (*contd.*)

Study	Country/Period	Sample	Drug	Crude overdose mortality rate per 1000	Proportion of deaths due to overdose (%)
Langendam et al. (2001)	Holland, 1985–1996	Treatment/community	Heroin, cocaine	6.3	21
Logan et al. (1998)	USA 1993–1995	Coronial	Amphetamine	n/a	36
Marx et al. (1994)	Switzerland 1987–1989	Drug-related deaths	Primarily opioids	n/a	86
Maxwell et al. (2005)	USA 1994–2002	Deaths in methadone	Opioids	n/a	14
McAnulty et al. (1995)	USA 1989–1991	Not in treatment	IDU	4.1	39
Miotto et al. (1997)	USA time unspecified	Treatment	Heroin	–	75
Musto & Ramos (1981)	USA 1918–1981	Treatment	Morphine	0.0	0
O'Doherty & Farrington (1997)	UK 1986–1991	Opioid deaths	Opioids	n/a	80
Oppenheimer et al. (1994)	UK 1969–1991	Treatment	Heroin	6.4	43
Orti et al. (1996)	Spain 1985–1991	Treatment, Hospital	Opioids	10.9	36
Oyefesso et al. (1999b)	UK 1974–1993	Notified teenage addicts	Opioids	4.7	69
Perucci et al. (1991)	Italy 1980–1988	Treatment	Opioids	2.4	33
Quaglio et al. (2001)	Italy 1985–1998	Treatment	IDU	–	37
Raikos et al. (2002)	Greece 1998–2000	Coronial	MDMA	n/a	14
Rehm et al. (2005)	Switzerland 1994–2000	Treatment	Heroin	1.1	10
Robertson et al. (1994)	UK 1982–1993	GP	IDU	7.4	38

Study	Location and period	Setting	Drug	Rate	N
Rossow (1994)	Norway 1968–1992	Treatment	"Addicts"	24.0	26
Schifano et al. (2003a)	UK 1996–2002	Coronial	MDMA	n/a	27
Tunving (1988)	Sweden 1970–1984	Treatment	Opioids, amphetamine	6.7	56
Vaillant (1973)	USA 1952–1970	Treatment, males	Narcotics	3.5	43
Van Ameidjen et al. (1999a)	Holland 1985–1995	Treatment and community agencies	IDU	5.0	33
Van Haarstrecht et al. (1996)	Holland 1985–1993	Treatment, sexually transmitted disease (STD) patients	IDU	5.6	25
Vlahov et al. (2004)	USA 1988–2000	New onset IDU	IDU	5.2	16
Wahren et al. (1997)	Sweden 1971–1990	Hospitalised for drug dependence	Stimulants, opioids	0.9	6
Watterson et al. (1975)	USA 1970–1974	Treatment	Opioids	4.3	33
Webb et al. (2003)	UK 2000	Drug-related deaths	All	n/a	77
Wille (1981)	UK 1969–1979	Treatment	Heroin	8.6	58
Zador & Sunjic (2000)	Australia 1990–1995	Treatment	Heroin	–	44
Zaccarelli et al. (1994)	Italy 1985–1991	Treatment	IDU	5.5	24
Zanis & Woody (1998)	USA 1993–1994	Methadone	Heroin	11.8	67
Zhu et al. (2000)	Japan 1994–1998	Coronial	Amphetamine	n/a	27

It is estimated that the proportion of heroin overdoses that result in death lies in the range of 2–4% (Darke et al., 2003b). As such, fatal overdoses represent only a small proportion of the total number of overdose events. Non-fatal overdose is of clinical significance, as it is associated with a range of serious sequelae, including pulmonary oedema, bronchopneumonia, rhabdomyolysis, peripheral neuropathy, renal failure, cognitive impairment, and traumatic injuries sustained during overdose (Warner-Smith et al., 2001). Few studies have systematically studied non-fatal overdose. Lifetime opioid overdose histories range from one- to two-thirds, and more than a quarter report an overdose in a 12-month period (Table 4.2). Given these rates of "near misses", the fact that overdose mortality rates are so high is not surprising.

Very few studies have been conducted on non-fatal cocaine overdose (Table 4.2). In part, this reflects difficulties of definition. Whereas heroin overdose is indicated by a well-recognised diagnostic triad of signs (reduced level of consciousness, miosis, respiratory depression), cocaine overdose is less clearly defined. Cocaine toxicity may manifest as a variety of acute physical and psychological

Table 4.2. Non-fatal overdose histories of illicit drug users

Study	Country	Lifetime overdose %	Recent overdose %
Opiates			
Bennett & Higgins (1999)	UK	–	30 (1 year)
Darke et al. (1996a)	Australia	68	29 (1 year)
Darke & Ross (1997b)	Australia	61	25 (1 year)
Darke & Ross (2001)	Australia	66	–
Darke et al. (2005f)	Australia	54	24 (1 year)
McGregor et al. (1998)	Australia	48	11 (6 months)
Neale & Robertson (2005)	UK	49	12 (3 months)
Powis et al. (1999)	UK	38	–
Stewart et al. (2002)	UK	–	15 (3 months)
Ochoa et al. (2001)	USA	48	–
Seal et al. (2001)	USA	48	13 ("recent")
Warner-Smith et al. (2003)	Australia	69	28 (1 year)
Cocaine			
Kaye & Darke (2004)	Australia	13	7 (1 year)
Pottieger et al. (1992)	USA	40	4 (3 months)
Mesquita et al. (2001)	Brazil	20	9 (2 years)
GHB			
Degenhardt et al. (2003)	Australia	53	–

symptoms, and does not necessarily entail loss of consciousness. Symptoms of cocaine overdose include nausea and vomiting, chest pain, tremors, increased body temperature, increased heart rate, breathing irregularities, and seizures (Karch, 2002). Lifetime overdose histories have ranged from 13% to 40% in published studies (Table 4.2). Whilst recent overdose rates are lower than amongst opiate users, they still constitute a significant proportion of cocaine users.

No study of non-fatal MDMA overdose has yet been published. The only published study of non-fatal overdose from a "party drug" examined GHB, a central nervous system (CNS) depressant that produces sedation and anaesthesia (Degenhardt et al., 2003). Approximately half of users reported having overdosed whilst using the drug, with overdose defined as loss of consciousness with an inability to be roused. This high figure indicates the potential for mortality amongst users of this drug, as use of the drug by the sample was a relatively recent phenomenon.

4.3   Demography of overdose

4.3.1   Opioids

Males constitute the overwhelming bulk of fatal opioid overdose cases, over 80% in some studies (e.g. Darke et al., 2000; Davidson et al., 2003; Fugelstad et al., 2003; Hickman et al., 2003; McGregor et al., 2002; Preti et al., 2002). An excess of male overdose cases is not surprising, given the over-representation of males among heroin users throughout the world. Whilst males represent approximately two-thirds of opiate users, however, they constitute a substantially higher proportion of overdose fatalities. As with illicit opioids, males also constitute the bulk of deaths attributed to both methadone and buprenorphine (Boyd et al., 2003; Bryant et al., 2004; Gagajewski & Apple, 2003; Kintz, 2001; Perret et al., 2000; Pirnay et al., 2004; Reynaud et al., 1998; Seymour et al., 2003; Sunjic & Zador, 1997; Tracqui et al., 1998; Williamson et al., 1997; Zador & Sunjic, 2000, 2002).

One of the most popular misconceptions regarding opioid overdose is that it is younger, inexperienced heroin users who are at greatest risk. As discussed in Chapter 3, however, the average age of death of opioid users is around 30 years. Not surprisingly, given the large proportion of illicit drug users who die from opioid overdose, the mean age of opioid overdose fatalities is also typically in the late 20s to early 30s (Darke et al., 2000; Davidson et al., 2003; Hickman et al., 2003). The age profile of case of deaths from methadone or buprenorphine toxicity are similar to those of heroin (Gagajewski & Apple, 2003; Perret et al.,

2000; Pirnay et al., 1998; Seymour et al., 2003; Sunjic & Zador, 1997; Williamson et al., 1997; Zador & Sunjic, 2002).

It is of particular clinical significance that heroin overdose cases are rarely in drug treatment at the time of overdose (Darke et al., 2000; Davidson et al., 2003; Davoli et al., 1993; Fugelstad et al., 1995; Perucci et al., 1991). These findings are important in informing attempts to reduce the rate of opioid overdose fatalities (cf. Chapter 8). While they are maintenance drugs, it should not be assumed that all deaths due to methadone or buprenorphine toxicity occur in treatment. Significant proportions of deaths from both drugs occur in persons who are not enrolled in a maintenance programme at the time of death, indicating diversion to the non-treatment population (Gagajewski & Apple, 2003; Kintz, 2001; Perret et al., 2000; Pirnay et al., 2004; Reynaud et al., 1998; Seymour et al., 2003; Sunjic & Zador, 1997; Zador & Sunjic, 2002).

4.3.2   Cocaine

As with opioid overdose, males constitute the bulk of fatal cocaine toxicity cases (Coffin et al., 2003; Darke et al., 2005a; Sanchez et al., 1995; Tardiff et al., 1996). To an extent, this also reflects the preponderance of males amongst illicit drug users. However, males are again over-represented, even after taking this into account, comprising over 80% of cases in some studies (Coffin et al., 2003; Darke et al., 2005a). Possible reasons for this over-representation are discussed below.

As with fatal opioid cases, deaths are not typically seen amongst young, inexperienced cocaine users, with the average age of decedents in the mid-30s (Coffin et al., 2003; Darke et al., 2005a; Sanchez et al., 1995; Tardiff et al., 1996). Again, these are older, experienced drug users, and not neophytes.

4.3.3   Amphetamines

There is not a large literature on the demographics of fatal amphetamine cases. As with both opioids and cocaine, males appear to dominate (Davis & Swalwell, 1994; Karch et al., 1999). In the largest reported series, males constituted 85% of cases (Karch et al., 1999). This clinical picture also appears true of survivors of amphetamine-induced acute cardiac infarction (Costa et al., 2001; Derlet et al., 1989; Farnsworth et al., 1997; Waksman et al., 2001). Again the typical clinical picture among fatalities is of older, experienced drug users (Hong et al., 1991; Karch et al.,1999; Ragland et al.,1993; Zhu et al., 2000). The mean age of cases in Karch et al. (1999) was 37 years, and the majority of cases of survivors of

amphetamine-induced acute cardiac infarction are older than 30 (Costa et al., 2001; Derlet et al., 1989; Waksman et al., 2001; Wijetunga et al., 2004).

4.3.4 MDMA

While there is substantially less data on deaths due to acute MDMA toxicity, males constitute the overwhelming majority of cases (Gill et al., 2002; Gowing et al., 2002; Lora-Tamayo et al., 1997; Schifano, 2004; Schifano et al., 2003a, b). In the UK, 80% of cases are male (Schifano et al., 2003a), and males constituted 75% of New York deaths (Gill et al., 2002). Data is scant, but the average age of death appears to be in the late 20s (Gill et al., 2002; Lora-Tamayo et al., 1997; Schifano et al., 2003a, b). There do, however, appear to be comparatively more younger cases (late teens to early 20s) than typically seen amongst opiate, cocaine, or amphetamine fatalities (Gill et al., 2002; Gowing et al., 2002). For instance, the mean age of the individual case reports reviewed by Gill et al. (2002) was only 22 years.

4.4 Mechanisms of overdose

4.4.1 Opioids

Heroin (diacetylmorphine) is rapidly hydrolysed to 6-monoacetylmorphine, which in turn is hydrolysed to morphine following administration in humans (Hardman et al., 1996). The clinical significance of morphine is that it is a CNS depressant, and respiration in humans is dependent upon CNS input. The primary mechanism of death in opioid overdose is thus opioid-induced depression of respiration, resulting in hypoxia and death (White & Irvine, 1999). Death from other opioid agonists, such as methadone, also result from respiratory depression. As noted above, the cardinal signs of heroin toxicity include reduced level of consciousness, pinpoint pupils, and a depressed respiratory rate. Cyanosis, hypotension, bradycardia, and hypothermia may also be present (Hardman et al., 1996; White & Irvine, 1999). Unlike heroin and methadone, buprenorphine has both opioid agonist and antagonist properties, and consequently is believed to have a lower risk of overdose (Boyd et al., 2003).

4.4.2 Cocaine

The major clinical distinction between the opioids and cocaine regarding overdose is that cocaine is cardiotoxic (Karch, 2002). Whilst death from opioid overdose relates primarily to respiratory depression, death from cocaine toxicity is due primarily to myocardial ischaemia and infarction (Karch, 2002). Cocaine can cause myocardial ischaemia and infarction through increased myocardial oxygen demand, coronary artery vasoconstriction, and coronary thrombosis (Karch, 2002; Kontos et al., 2003; Lange & Hillis, 2001; Moliterno et al., 1994; Petitti et al., 1998).

Although cocaine can induce cardiovascular complications in users with normal coronary arteries (Lange & Hillis, 2001; Vasica & Tennant, 2002), underlying atherosclerosis (particularly of the left anterior descending coronary artery) has been consistently demonstrated (Darke et al., 2005a; Hollander et al., 1997; Karch, 2002; Kontos et al., 2003; Mittleman et al., 1999; Vasica & Tennant, 2002). Such premature and accelerated coronary artery atherosclerosis, increases the risk of cocaine-induced myocardial infarction. Chronic cocaine use had also been associated with left ventricular hypertrophy, due to increased myocardial oxygen demands, a condition that also predisposes to myocardial ischaemia and/or arrhythmia (Karch, 2002; Om et al., 1993).

Consistent with the cardiotoxic profile of cocaine, chest pains and palpitations are among the most common complaints among cocaine users presenting with acute cocaine toxicity (Kaye & Darke, 2005; Kontos et al., 2003; Lange & Hillis, 2001). Cocaine-induced cerebrovascular accident is also well recognised as a cause of death (Karch, 2002). A recent study demonstrated a 14-fold increase in risk of ischaemic or haemorrhagic stroke among cocaine users compared to matched controls (Pettiti et al., 1998).

4.4.3   *Amphetamines*

As with cocaine, amphetamine is a stimulant that places demands upon the cardiovascular system, increasing heart rate, and blood pressure (Perez-Reyes et al., 1991). More particularly, amphetamine is also known to be cardiotoxic (Karch, 2002), Indeed, the pathological effects of amphetamine are similar to, or indistinguishable from, those attributable to cocaine (Julien, 2001; Sztajnkryeer, 2002). The primary long-term effect of amphetamine use is also accelerated development of coronary artery disease, particularly atherosclerotic stenosis or occlusion (Karch 2002; Karch et al., 1999, Kaye & McKetin, 2005; Logan et al., 1998; Wijetunga et al., 2004). Other documented pathological effects of amphetamine include myocardial infarction/ischaemia, cardiomyopathy, cardiac hypertrophy, sudden acute aortic dissection, and cardiac vasospasm (Karch, 2002; Karch et al., 1999; Swalwell & Davis, 1999; Wijetunga et al., 2003; Zhu et al., 2000). As with cocaine, coronary vasospasm may occur where there is no underlying coronary artery disease (Lange & Hillis, 2001). Consistent with the pathological effects of amphetamine, chest pains, palpitation, tachycardia, and hypertension are the most common presenting symptoms in emergency departments relating to acute amphetamine intoxication (Lan et al., 1998; Richards et al., 1999; Turnispeed et al., 2003).

As would be expected, given this clinical profile, amphetamine-induced cerebrovascular accident has been well documented (Davis & Swalwell, 1994; Karch, 2002; Karch et al., 1999; Zhu et al., 2000). Pettiti et al. (1998) found a 4-fold increase in the risk of ischaemic or haemorrhagic stroke among amphetamine users compared to controls.

While both cocaine and amphetamine are distinguishable from opioids in that both are cardiotoxic, the incidence of serious pathological effects of amphetamine appears less common than those associated with cocaine (Derlet & Horowitz, 1995; Karch, 2002; Petitti et al., 1998; Wijetunga et al., 2004). While, for example, the elevated risk of cerebrovascular accident reported by Pettiti et al. (1998) was 4-fold for amphetamine, the corresponding figure for cocaine was 14-fold. This may explain why cocaine constitutes a larger proportion of overdose fatalities than does amphetamine (e.g. Coffin et al., 2003), despite the widespread use of amphetamine. This observation must, however, be tempered by the fact that substantially less research has been conducted into amphetamine-related death than is the case with cocaine.

4.4.4 MDMA

There are a number of mechanisms that may result in death from acute MDMA toxicity, including hyperthermia, cerebral oedema due to excess water consumption, cardiovascular complications, and liver failure. The most commonly identified acute reaction to MDMA is hyperthermia (Gowing et al., 2002; Schifano, 2004). After MDMA administration, the core body temperature may rise to more than 42°C. Such temperatures may result in collapse, coma, seizure, rhabdomyolysis (muscle breakdown), liver impairment, and kidney failure. To an extent, the fact that MDMA is commonly taken in nightclubs with high ambient temperatures, and that the person may be constantly exerting themselves, exacerbates this syndrome. It is important to recognise, however, that hyperthermia may be a direct effect of the drug itself, and can occur in quiet surroundings (Gowing et al., 2002).

A second mechanism is excessive water consumption (Gowing et al., 2002; Karch, 2002; Schifano, 2004). This may result in death from hyponatraemia (decreased sodium concentrations) or from cerebral oedema. Excess water consumption may be due to sweating (due to high core and ambient temperatures), as well as physical activity. MDMA, however, also appears to produce sensations of thirst, independent of actual need (Gowing et al., 2002). The antidiuretic effects of MDMA also contribute to the syndrome.

As an amphetamine-like stimulant, MDMA has similar effects upon the cardiovascular and cerebrovascular systems. Whilst apparently not the most common mechanism of death, there are documented cases of death from cardiac arrest, aortic dissection, and cerebral ischaemia (DuFlou & Mark, 2000; Gowing et al., 2002; Karch, 2002). Clearly, the presence of pre-existing cardiac or cerebrovascular disease, and/or excessive exertion in dance clubs, would exacerbate such risk.

Finally, MDMA appears to have direct hepatotoxic effects, and may directly cause liver failure (Gowing et al., 2002; Karch, 2002; Selim & Kaplowitz, 1999). Whilst most cases of liver damage have arisen as a result of hyperthermia, there are cases where severe liver damage has occurred in the absence of hyperthermia (Gowing et al., 2002).

4.5   Toxicology of overdose

4.5.1   Opioids

The classical depiction of a fatal heroin "overdose", as the result of a quantity or quality (purity) of heroin in excess of the person's current tolerance to the drug, is the most long-standing explanation for death. Morphine concentrations in fatal cases, however, have been consistently skewed towards the lower end of the range (e.g. Darke et al., 2000; Fugelstad et al., 2003; Gerostamoulos et al., 2001; Kintz et al., 1989; Kronstrand et al., 1998; Monforte, 1977). Indeed, direct comparisons indicate that fatal overdose cases are likely to have morphine levels no higher than overdose survivors or living intoxicated heroin users (Aderjan et al., 1995; Darke et al., 1997; Gutierrez-Cebollada et al., 1994; Monforte, 1977).

Fluctuations in heroin purity also appear to have only a moderate relationship to the incidence of heroin-related death. As long ago as the 1970s, Desmond et al. (1978) in the US, reported no correlation between heroin potency and overdose fatalities. Ruttenber & Luke (1984), found heroin purity accounted for only a quarter of the variance in overdose fatalities, as did Darke et al. (1999), while Risser et al. (2000) found no relationship between the purity of heroin seizures and heroin-related death.

Some studies have reported the presence of contaminants, usually quinine, in heroin samples or the blood of decedents (Cherubin et al., 1972; Monforte,

1977; Ruttenber & Luke, 1984). In general, however, harmful contaminants have been rarely detected outside the eastern US, and those that were typically relatively innocuous substances, such as sucrose (Coomber, 1997, 1999; Maher et al., 2001). More broadly, contaminants play no role in deaths from methadone or buprenorphine. Overall there is no toxicological evidence that contaminants play a major role in opioid overdose.

Possibly the most important finding to emerge in recent years is that the overwhelming majority of heroin overdoses involve the concomitant consumption of heroin with other drugs (Darke et al., 2000; Davidson et al., 2003; Fugelstad et al., 2003; Gerostamoulos et al., 2001; Hickman et al., 2003; McGregor et al., 2002; Preti et al., 2002). The major drugs involved are alcohol, benzodiazepines, tricyclic antidepressants, and cocaine. Importantly, concomitant polydrug use also extends to deaths attributed to methadone and buprenorphine (Boyd et al., 2003; Bryant et al., 2004; Hickman et al., 2003; Kintz, 2001; Perret et al., 2000; Pirnay et al., 2004; Reynaud et al., 1998; Seymour et al., 2003; Zador & Sunjic, 2000).

By far the most common concomitant drug detected is alcohol, typically present in half or more of cases (Darke et al., 2000; Davidson et al., 2003; Fugelstad et al., 2003; Gerostamoulos et al., 2001; Hickman et al., 2003; McGregor et al., 2002; Preti et al., 2002). There is an inverse relationship between blood morphine and alcohol concentrations, with lower morphine concentrations detected in the presence of alcohol (Darke et al., 2000; Fugelstad et al., 2003; Ruttenber & Luke, 1984; Ruttenber et al., 1990). Benzodiazepines are also noted in up to quarter of cases (Caplehorn, 1996; Davidson et al., 2003; Fugelstad et al., 2003; Gerostamoulos et al., 2001). In fact, there is evidence of an increase in the frequency of benzodiazepine prescriptions in the weeks preceding death (Burns et al., 2004; Martyres et al., 2004). The role of alcohol and benzodiazepines are not restricted to heroin overdose, with both drugs strongly associated with methadone and buprenorphine deaths (Boyd et al., 2003; Bryant et al., 2004; Hickman et al., 2003; Kintz, 2001; Perret et al., 2000; Pirnay et al., 2004; Reynaud et al., 1998; Seymour et al., 2003; Zador & Sunjic, 2000).

Antidepressants use, and tricyclic antidepressant use in particular, has also been linked to opiate overdose, present in up to a tenth of cases (Darke et al., 2000; Martyres et al., 2004). Finally, cocaine is commonly detected, particularly in the US (Coffin et al., 2003; Darke et al., 2000; Davidson et al., 2003; Tardiff et al., 1996). A quarter of heroin overdoses in San Francisco also had cocaine detected (Davidson et al., 2003), as did nearly a tenth of Australian cases, where cocaine use is substantially less common (Darke et al., 2000).

4.5.2   Cocaine

While cocaine dose and frequency of use may influence the likelihood of coronary and cerebrovascular complications, the threshold over which potentially fatal reactions occur varies widely between individuals. Toxic reactions can occur irrespective of dose, frequency of use, or route of administration, and have been reported with small amounts of cocaine and on the first occasion of use (Karch, 2002; Lange & Hillis, 2001; Platt, 1997). Overall there appears to be no well-delineated dose response for cocaine toxicity (Karch et al., 1998; Karch, 2002; Lange & Hillis, 2001).

As with opioid overdose, multiple drugs are typically detected among cocaine-related fatalities, most commonly heroin in over half of cases, and alcohol in over a fifth (Coffin et al., 2003; Darke et al., 2005a; Tardiff et al., 1996; Wetli & Wright, 1979). Tricyclic antidepressants were also reported in nearly one in ten cases (Darke et al., 2005a; Tardiff et al., 1996). The role of polydrug use is illustrated by Coffin et al. (2003). Changes in both cocaine and heroin overdoses rates were related to changes in the rate of polydrug deaths, whilst the rate of single drug deaths remained stable. Similarly, non-fatal cocaine overdose has been strongly related to concomitant drug use (Kaye & Darke, 2004). Toxic contaminants are not widely found amongst cocaine fatalites (Darke et al., 2005a; Tardiff et al., 1996).

4.5.3   Amphetamines

As with cocaine, toxic reactions to amphetamine can occur irrespective of dose, frequency of use, or route of administration, and even small doses have been known to cause death (Fukunaga et al., 1987; Karch, 2002; Karch et al., 1989; Zhu et al., 2000). Again, as with cocaine, there appears to be no well-delineated dose response for amphetamine toxicity. Indeed, blood methamphetamine concentrations reported in Karch et al. (1999) were not significantly different from those of cases where methamphetamine was the cause of death.

It is difficult to determine the role of polydrug use in amphetamine toxicity cases, as little data are available. Where multiple toxicology has been reported, multiple substances were detected in approximately half of cases, most commonly alcohol (10–25%), cocaine (12–25%), and morphine (20–30%) (Karch et al., 1999; Logan et al., 1998). There is no evidence that contaminants play a significant role in these deaths (Karch et al., 1999; Logan et al., 1998; Shaw, 1999; Zhu et al., 2000).

4.5.4 MDMA

Like the two stimulants discussed above, there appears to be no well-defined dose response for MDMA toxicity (Gowing et al., 2002; Karch, 2002; Schifano, 2004). In fact, in a finding that appears to be common across drug classes, blood MDMA concentrations in fatal cases have been demonstrated to be no higher than those of others who died from unrelated causes (Gill et al., 2002).

As with other forms of drug-related death, multiple drugs typically are detected in fatal MDMA cases (Gill et al., 2002; Gowing et al., 2002; Lora-Tamayo et al., 1997; Schifano et al., 2003a, b). The most commonly reported other drugs have been alcohol, amphetamine, cocaine, and opiates. The largest series (Schifano et al., 2003a) reported other drugs in over 80% of cases: alcohol (19%), amphetamine (12%), cocaine (13%), and opiates (27%). While most deaths involve multiple substances it is important to note, given its image as a safe drug, that MDMA by itself is involved in a significant proportion of cases. As with other drugs, there is no evidence that contaminants play a significant role (Gill et al., 2002; Schifano, 2004).

4.6 Risk factors for overdose

Risk factors for overdose fall into five broad areas: demographic characteristics, polydrug use, drug purity, drug tolerance, and route of administration (Table 4.3). Whilst some of these factors have been discussed earlier in this chapter when describing the dynamics of overdose, a more discursive analysis follows.

4.6.1 Demographics

4.6.1.1 Age

As noted earlier, it is older users who constitute the bulk of heroin overdose deaths. This is puzzling as such a population would be expected to have a high tolerance. One possible explanation is that it simply reflects cumulative risk exposure. If it is assumed that each instance of heroin administration is associated with a discrete risk of overdose, cumulative risk will increase on each successive administration. The analogy here is with Russian roulette, with the overall age profile a consequence of repeated risk episodes. The fact that methadone and buprenorphine fatalities are also typically older may reflect the fact that larger proportions of these cases were enrolled in treatment (Perret et al., 2000; Reynaud et al., 1998; Seymour et al., 2003; Sunjic & Zador, 1997; Williamson

Table 4.3. Factors associated with overdose

Variable	Comment
Demographics	
Gender	Overwhelmingly male
Age	Mean age in early 30s. More younger cases for MDMA
Dependence	Long-term dependent users predominate
Treatment status	Rarely enrolled in treatment
Tolerance	
Heroin	Possible reduced heroin use prior to death in many cases
Cocaine, amphetamine, MDMA	No strong dose response
Prison	Post-release period high risk of opioid overdose
Purity	
Purity level	Only moderately related to heroin overdose
Contaminants	Harmful contaminants rarely detected
Polydrug use	
Alcohol	Strong association with opioid and cocaine deaths. Possible link to amphetamine and MDMA
Benzodiazepines	Increased risk of opioid overdose
Tricyclic antidepressants	Increased risk of heroin and cocaine overdose
Cocaine + heroin	Increased risk of overdose
Amphetamine + cocaine	Increased risk of overdose
Route of administration	
Injecting	Substantially increases risk of overdose for opiates, cocaine, and amphetamine
Smoking/oral/nasal	Reduced risk of heroin overdose. High proportions of cocaine and amphetamine fatalities

et al., 1997). Cases not in treatment may well also be a reflection of the cumulative risk.

An alternative, though not incompatible, explanation relates to the natural history of heroin use. Two recent studies (Darke et al., 2002; Tagliaro et al., 1998) reported hair morphine concentrations among fatal overdose cases were significantly lower than those of current users, indicating less frequent heroin use in the period immediately prior to death. Similarly, a recent study found no hair morphine in a third of fatal overdose cases (Kronstrand et al., 1998), while Fugeslstad et al. (2003) reported a quarter of fatal cases had periods of abstinence immediately prior to death. How does this relate to the natural history of drug use? The rigours of the heroin lifestyle may mean that, after a decade or so of heroin use, many users cut down their use. They may also increase their use of other drugs, such as alcohol and benzodiazepines, to compensate for their reduced heroin use (Burns et al., 2004; Fugeslstad et al., 2003; Martyres et al., 2004). The low blood morphine concentrations detected in many fatal overdose cases may thus reflect less frequent use, and correspondingly lower tolerance to opioids, among older heroin users.

The older age profile of cocaine-related fatalities may also simply reflect the cumulative risk exposure of repeated use. The effects of repeated cocaine administration are, however, quite distinct from those seen in the use of opioids. As discussed previously, repeated cocaine administration results in cumulative risk of cardiac and coronary artery disease, most commonly ventricular hypertrophy and atherosclerosis. The accumulated damage from long-term cocaine use may substantially increase risk of myocardial infarction as the user ages, and substantially increase the risk for each individual use episode over time. This argument clearly also applies to amphetamine-related fatalities, who are also typically older, longer-term users (Hong et al., 1991; Huang et al., 2003; Karch et al., 1999; Waksman et al., 2001; Zhu et al., 2000).

The possibly younger profile of recreational MDMA user deaths may reflect the fact that the primary cause of such death is hyperthermia. It is younger people who are more likely to attend dance parties, with high ambient temperatures, and to engage in excessive exertions. In this, MDMA may be more like opioids, where rather than cumulative damage, it is situational risk that is of importance.

4.6.1.2 Gender

Being male is a clear risk factor for overdose death. Why are males over-represented in opioid, cocaine, and amphetamine overdose fatalities, even allowing for the dominance of males in drug-using populations? Two possible factors that have emerged from the heroin literature are the higher rates of alcohol use seen among male overdose cases, and the greater social isolation of male users. Specifically, it has been reported that male heroin users are more likely to be alcohol dependent than females (Darke & Ross, 1997a), and that male overdose fatalities are more likely to have alcohol detected (Darke et al., 2000). The excess of male cases may thus be due to their higher rates of concomitant alcohol use, which substantially increases their risk of overdose from heroin, as well as methadone, and buprenorphine. Male heroin users are also less likely to be married, or to live with others, than are females (Davoli et al., 1993). As such, they are more likely to be alone at the time of an overdose, increasing their risk of death.

The preponderance of male cocaine and amphetamine fatalities may well reflect the fact that there are substantially higher rates of cardiac disease amongst males in the general population. Males are more prone to cardiac disease, and the use of a cardiotoxic drug that places heavy demands upon the cardiovascular system may differentially increase the risk to male users. Apart from a similar higher risk for MDMA-induced cardiac arrest or cerebrovascular accident, it is unclear why males constitute such a high proportion of MDMA fatalities.

4.6.1.3   *Treatment*

The third major demographic factor involved in overdose deaths is that overdoses cases from all drug classes are not frequently in treatment at the time of death (Darke et al., 2000, 2005a; Davidson et al., 2003; Karch et al., 1999; Schifano, 2004). In part, this reflects the overall success of drug-treatment programmes in reducing the frequency of illicit drug use. Users in treatment are using their primary drug of dependence far less frequently, or not using at all, and are thus at a substantially lower risk of overdose. Consistent with this, treatment for opiate dependence has been demonstrated to reduce the risk of non-fatal heroin overdose (Darke et al., 2005f; Stewart et al., 2003). Moreover, in the case of opioid substitution treatments, high opioid tolerance is maintained by the regular administration of a long-acting opioid, reducing the risk of overdose if illicit drug use continues.

4.6.2   *Tolerance*

The very term "overdose" implies that death is due to variations in drug purity exceeding the drug tolerance of individuals. The demographic characteristics and the toxicology of overdose cases has, however, thrown doubt on this simple explanation, and suggest that overdose is a great deal more complicated than a simple exceeding of tolerance. This is not to say that tolerance is not a relevant factor. Evidence that many cases had reduced their use prior to death implies a loss of tolerance in these individuals. More broadly, it has recently been proposed that the natural history of tolerance development may partially explain why so many cases occur amongst older users (White & Irvine, 1999). Specifically, it has been proposed that tolerance to the hedonistic effects of opioids develops more rapidly than tolerance to the respiratory effects, with the later being an incomplete tolerance (White & Irvine, 1999). As the heroin use career progresses, the ratio between the dose that is needed to obtain the required effects and that which is lethal decreases. Effectively, the safety margin between the amount needed to obtain euphoric effects and that required to cease respiration diminishes. Given this, it is longer-term heroin users who would be expected to suffer overdoses.

In addition to general risk, there are specific situations in which opioid tolerance is clearly a major issue. In particular, the period immediately post-prison release constitutes a high risk for overdose among heroin users (Seaman et al., 1998; Seymour et al., 2000). Whilst many heroin users continue to inject in prison, such use is typically sporadic, resulting in substantially reduced tolerance. A similar situation exists where use is resumed after maintenance on the opioid antagonist naltrexone (Digiusto et al., 2004; Miotto et al., 1997; Oliver et al., 2005), and with the period immediately following a successful opioid detoxification (Strang et al., 2003). Finally, the induction phase of methadone maintenance represents a period where the risk of methadone overdose is highest, and prescribed dosages may exceed tolerance (Buster et al., 2002; Zador & Sunjic, 2002). Finally, the period immediately after the cessation of treatment constitutes a high-risk period for overdose (Davoli et al., 1993; Fugelstad et al., 2003; Gronbladh et al., 1990).

The absence of a well-documented dose response for cocaine toxicity is believed to be due to its cardiotoxic effects (Karch, 2002; Karch et al., 1998; Lange & Hillis, 2001). The cumulative cardiotoxic effects of cocaine may produce cardiopathology, after which even small amounts of cocaine may result in death. Low cocaine blood concentrations have also been shown to produce acute vasospasm, which may induce myocardial infarction or ischaemia (Karch, 2002; Lange & Hillis, 2001; Moliterno et al., 1994). Clearly, the similar cardiotoxic effects of amphetamine mean that similar arguments apply to this drug (Karch, 2002). Indeed, in cases where amphetamine-related cardiac disease is present, post-mortem toxicology may reveal very low amphetamine concentrations (Karch, 2002).

Reasons for the similar absence of a clear dose response to MDMA concentrations are unclear. Given the primary mechanisms of death discussed above (hyperthermia, excessive water consumption, cardiac toxicity), possible explanations for these findings include individual differences in susceptibility to hyperthermia, pre-existing cardiac disease, differences in water consumption, and differences in exertions due to setting (Gowing et al., 2002).

4.6.3 *Purity*

As noted previously, variations in heroin purity only moderately relate to the incidence of heroin overdose. A general increase in heroin purity will, in all likelihood, produce only moderate increases in overdose death rates. The implication is that there are other factors involved that ameliorate the role of drug purity. Two findings from the literature are relevant. First, the majority of cases occur amongst older, dependent heroin users, most of whom would presumably be tolerant to all but extreme variations in purity. This does not, of course apply to those who have reduced their use. Second, other drugs, which substantially increase the risk of overdose, are involved in the majority of overdose cases. Overdose cases are thus not simply related to a single drug. If multiple drug use is a major factor, variations in concomitant drug use may play a larger role than variations in purity. Indeed, as noted, Coffin et al. (2003) reported that variations in multiple drug deaths were strongly related to the overall incidence of heroin deaths.

To date, there are no epidemiological studies of the relationship between drug purity, and cocaine-, amphetamine-, or MDMA-related deaths.

4.6.4   Polydrug use

As discussed above, multiple drugs are typically reported in fatal opioid overdose cases. Is this merely an artefact, or are there pharmacological reasons why such concomitant drug use may contribute to death? Alcohol and benzodiazepines, the most commonly detected drugs are, like heroin and other opioids, CNS depressants. It is likely that there is potentiation of the respiratory depressant effects of these drugs when taken with heroin. Thus, in the presence of other CNS depressant drugs a usual dose of heroin may well prove fatal, due to the combined depressant effects of these drugs. The fact that negative correlations between morphine and ethanol concentrations are frequently reported is consistent with this view (Darke et al., 2000; Fugelstad et al., 2003; Ruttenber & Luke, 1984; Ruttenber et al., 1990). Indeed, it would be surprising if the concomitant use of CNS depressant did *not* increase risk of death when using opioids. Clearly, the same argument applies to the fact that alcohol and benzodiazepines are also strongly associated with death from methadone and buprenorphine. In the latter case, they may well play a more clinically significantly role, given the innate opioid antagonist properties of buprenorphine.

Risk of heroin overdose would appear to be increased by tricyclic antidepressant use, but *not* selective serotonin reuptake inhibitor (SSRI) use (Darke & Ross, 2000a; Martyres et al., 2004). The link is thus likely to be pharmacological, rather than antidepressants merely being a proxy for depression, and suicide (cf. Chapter 6). Given that the major toxic effects of tricyclic antidepressant drugs include coma, convulsions respiratory depression and cardiac arrest (Dziukas & Vohra, 1991), a relationship to opioid overdose should not surprise.

The combination of cocaine and heroin appears to be more dangerous than using either drug alone. It has been hypothesised that cocaine may potentiate the tendency of opioids to depress respiration (Jaffe, 1985; Platt, 1997; Polettini et al., 2005). It may also be speculated that respiratory depression may induce cardiac failure among cases where cardiac disease is present. Thus, while opioids depress respiration, there is a contiguous increased myocardial oxygen demand due to the effects of cocaine.

Like opioid overdose, there is a strong association between alcohol and cocaine overdose. The reasons for this association, however, differ from the association between opioids and alcohol. The concomitant ingestion of cocaine and alcohol produces cocaethylene, an active metabolite of cocaine which is not only more toxic than cocaine itself, but which has a synergistic effect in increasing the toxicity of cocaine (Brookoff et al., 1996; Harris et al., 2003; Karch, 2002). Increased risk here is thus due to the production of a *third* psychoactive substance, rather than their interaction *per se*.

The fact that tricyclic antidepressants have been associated with cocaine overdose deaths (Darke et al., 2005a; Tardiff et al., 1996) in all probability reflects the known cardiotoxicity of both tricyclic antidepressants and cocaine. Such a combination would be likely to increase the risk of myocardial infarction.

As discussed previously, there is not an extensive literature upon which to base firm conclusions about the role of polydrug use in amphetamine-related death. The two most likely drugs implicated, however, are alcohol and cocaine. When amphetamine is combined with alcohol or cocaine or opiates, toxicity is increased (Albertson et al., 1999; Mendelson et al., 1995). Unlike cocaine, the combination of alcohol and amphetamine does not produce a new psychoactive substance. The combination does, however, increase heart rate and blood pressure beyond that seen for amphetamine alone (Mendelson et al., 1995). As would be expected, combining amphetamine and cocaine has been demonstrated to substantially increase the vasoconstrictive and cardiotoxic effects of amphetamine (Welder, 1992). Given the cardiotoxic effects of amphetamine, it is reasonable to speculate that the concomitant use of alcohol or cocaine may increase the risk of toxic reactions. The presence of morphine in amphetamine overdose cases, like cocaine, may be due to the fact that while opioids depress respiration, there is a contiguous increased myocardial oxygen demand due to the effects of amphetamine.

As discussed above, polydrug use is common amongst MDMA fatalities. In the case of opiates, there is no obvious mechanism of interaction with MDMA.

Alcohol, however, has been demonstrated to increase the physiopathological effects of MDMA (Schifano, 2004). Concomitant use of other stimulants, such as cocaine or amphetamine, may well exacerbate risk, as they would be expected to increase the risk of cardiac arrest and/or cerebrovascular accident. On a behavioural level, it is possible that they may increase overall arousal and exertion, although this is speculative.

4.6.5   *Route of administration*

In recent years the smoking of heroin, or more properly its inhalation, has become widespread (Strang et al., 1997). Most commonly the drug is heated on aluminium foil, and the vapours inhaled through a tube, a process known as "chasing the dragon" or simply "chasing". Overdose risk appears to be substantially lower when the drug is smoked, rather than injected (Brugal et al., 2005; Carpenter et al., 1998; Darke et al., 2005b; Swift et al., 1999). Lower risk levels are thought to be due to the titration of doses involved, in which small amounts are smoked sequentially, compared to injecting where a morphine bolus is delivered to the brain. Whilst heroin injecting appears to involve substantially greater risk, it is important to emphasise that death can result from non-injecting routes (Darke & Ross, 2000b; Thiblin et al., 2004).

It is important to note that significant proportions of deaths from methadone syrup and buprenorphine had injected the drug prior to death (Boyd et al., 2003; Kintz, 2001; Perret et al., 2000; Pirnay et al., 2004; Reynaud et al., 1998; Sunjic & Zador, 1997). The injection of a long-acting oral preparation would be expected to increase the risk of death, due to the higher blood concentrations being delivered to the brain compared to oral administration.

The likelihood of a cocaine overdose also increases when cocaine is administered in a way that causes a rapid increase in blood and brain levels of the drug, increasing risk of seizure, stroke, cardiac arrest, or respiratory arrest. Injecting cocaine is likely to pose the greatest risk of overdose, followed by smoking and intranasal use (Kaye & Darke, 2004; Karch, 2002; Potteigger et al., 1992). Consistent with this, injectors are at greater risk of non-fatal cocaine overdose (Kaye & Darke, 2004; Mesquita et al., 2001; Potteiger et al., 1992), and they comprise the majority of fatal overdose cases (Darke et al., 2005a; Wetli & Wright, 1979). It is important to note, however, that whilst injecting may increase proximal risk, use by any route may result in the development of coronary artery atherosclerosis and left ventricular hypertrophy. Unlike the opioids, in which each use episode carries an independent risk, regular cocaine use by any means may cumulatively increase the likelihood of cardiac arrest.

This may partially explain why, in the few studies that have measured route of administration, there are higher proportions of non-injectors seen amongst cocaine fatalities than usually occurs amongst illicit opioid users (Darke et al., 2005a; Wetli & Wright, 1979).

There appears to be a high proportion of fatalities and near fatalities associated with non-injecting amphetamine administration (Farnsworth et al., 1997; Hong et al., 1991; Karch et al., 1999; Ragland et al., 1993; Zhu et al., 2000). Injectors, however, constitute a substantial proportions of cases. Karch et al. (1999) found evidence of injecting in a third of cases, while Zhu et al. (2000) reported all 15 amphetamine-related deaths in their study to show evidence of injection. Fatal and near fatal amphetamine-induced myocardial infarction has been reported, however, from oral administration, nasal administration, and smoking (Costa, 2001; Furst et al., 1990; Guharoy et al., 1999; Hong et al., 1991; Huang et al., 1993; Orzel, 1982; Wijetunga et al., 2003). As with cocaine, regular amphetamine use by any means may cumulatively increase the likelihood of cardiac arrest due to accumulated cardiovascular damage.

As an oral drug used in tablet form, and primarily by non-dependent recreational users, there is no evidence to date to indicate that injecting plays a significant role in MDMA-related death.

4.7   Summary of mortality and overdose

Overdose is a major cause of death amongst illicit drug using cohorts, and a risk not present among non-drug using populations. The mechanisms of overdose differ by drug class, although many issues surrounding overdose remain unresolved. Opioid fatalities are primarily due to respiratory depression, whilst deaths from psychostimulant drugs are primarily due to cardiovascular complications.

The demographic profile of overdose fatalities is predominantly male, aged in the early 30s, with extensive drug-using careers. Contrary to popular perception, it is not the young and inexperienced who are at greatest risk. Similarly, despite the term "overdose", blood concentrations of overdose cases are in many cases low, or similar to non-drug deaths. In the case of cocaine, amphetamine, and MDMA, there is no well-delineated dose response. The majority of overdose deaths involve combinations of drugs. The injection of illicit drugs carries the greatest risk of overdose, but fatalities occur from all routes of administration. The implications of the issues discussed in this chapter for both research priorities and interventions to reduce overdose-related mortality will be considered in Chapters 8 and 9.

Key points: Summary of overdose and illicit drug use

- Overdose deaths constitute more than a quarter of drug-related deaths in most studies.
- Overdose mortality exceed 5 per 10 thousand person years in most studies.
- Opioid overdoses are primarily due to respiratory depression, whilst cocaine and amphetamine toxicity is typically due to myocardial infarction or stroke. The major cause of MDMA deaths is hyperthermia.
- The "typical" overdose cases is male, in their early 30s, and not enrolled in drug treatment.
- The presence of a single drug at overdose is atypical.
- Variations in heroin purity are only moderately associated with overdose rates.
- Injection carries the greatest risk of overdose, but fatalities occur from all routes of administration.

5

Illicit drug use and disease

5.1 Introduction

This chapter will examine the major diseases associated with illicit drug use, and their contribution to mortality. As noted in Chapter 3, there are specific disease risks that are associated with illicit drug use that increase its salience as a cause of premature death. The impact that disease makes upon illicit drug using populations is illustrated in Table 5.1. In many of the studies of illicit drug user deaths conducted since the 1980s (after the advent of the human immunodeficiency virus (HIV) pandemic) the majority of the cohort have died as a result of disease, mostly commonly acquired immunodeficiency syndrome (AIDS) (Bargagli et al., 2001; Goedert et al., 1995; Langendam et al., 2001; Maxwell et al., 2005; Rehm et al., 2005; Zaccarelli et al., 1994).

In terms of the major diseases, drug injectors are at particular risk of infection with HIV or hepatitis C virus (HCV) through the sharing of injection equipment, and through unprotected sexual activity (in the case of HIV). HIV is a major cause of mortality among injecting drug users (IDU), as can clearly be seen in the studies presented in Table 5.1. Deaths related to chronic HCV infection may also constitute an increasingly important cause of mortality among this group. Infections such as endocarditis are also a risk for IDU if they use unsterile injecting equipment.

Given the mechanism of action of drugs such as cannabis, cocaine, and methamphetamine on the body, the risks to the cardiovascular system (and potential for death) will also be considered in this chapter.

5.2 HIV/AIDS

One of the most widely discussed causes of death among IDU is HIV/AIDS (cf. Table 5.1). In 2003, it was estimated that almost 38 million persons were

Table 5.1. Disease as a cause of death amongst illicit drug users

Study	Country/period	Sample	Drug	Crude disease mortality rate (per 1000 person years)	Proportion of deaths due to disease (AIDS)(%)
Bargagli et al. (2001)	Italy 1980–1997	Treatment	Heroin	11.6(8.4)	54(39)
Bartu et al. (2004)	Australia 1985–1998	Hospital/psych. admissions	Opioids, amphetamine	0.5(0.1)	30(4)
Benson & Holmberg (1984)	Sweden 1968–1978	Conscripts, rehab. & Psych. patients, welfare recipients	Cannabis, solvents, Lysergic acid diethylamine, stimulants	0.2(0)	5(0)
Bentley & Busuttil (1996)	UK 1989–1994	Coronial cases	Opioids	n/a	9(5)
Bewley et al. (1968)	UK 1947–1966	Notified addicts	Heroin	10.5(0)	39(0)
Brugal et al. (2005)	Spain 1992–1999	Treatment	Heroin	–(0.2)	–(38)
Bucknall & Robertson (1986)	UK 1981–1985	General practitioners (GP) attendees	Heroin	0(0)	0(0)
Caplehorn et al. (1996)	Australia 1979–1991	Treatment	Heroin	–(0)	–(0)
Cherubin et al. (1972)	US 1964–1968	Notified addicts	Heroin	–(–)	15(0)
Cooncool et al. (1979)	US 1969–1976	Treatment	Heroin	2.2(0)	40(0)
Davoli et al. (1997)	Italy 1980–1992	Treatment	IDU	12.0(10.6)	49(30)
Dukes et al. (1992)	New Zealand 1971–1989	Notified teenage addicts	Opioids	2.7(0)	37(0)
Engstrom et al. (1991)	Sweden 1973–1984	Drug-related hospitalisation	Amphetamine, cocaine, heroin	9.2(–)	40(–)
Eskild et al. (1993)	Norway 1985–1991	HIV test centre	IDU	1.6(1.1)	7(5)
Friedman et al. (1996)	US 1984–1992	Welfare recipients	Drugs and alcohol	14.2(10.2)	50(36)
Frischer et al. (1997)	UK 1982–1994	Treatment	IDU	5.2(0.4)	25(2)

Reference	Period	Sample	Drug		
Fugelstad et al. (1995)	Sweden 1986–1990	HIV + drug addicts	Heroin	9.6(3.9)	25(10)
Fugelstad et al. (1997)	Sweden 1981–1992	Drug-related hospitalisation	Heroin, amphetamine	3.1(1.4)	19(8)
Galli & Musicco (1994)	Italy 1980–1991	Treatment	Methadone	11.8(8.8)	47(35)
Gardner (1970)	UK 1965–1969	Coronial cases	Opioids	n/a	21(0)
Goedert et al. (1995)	Italy 1980–1990	Treatment	Heroin	11.5(7.1)	73(45)
Goldstein & Herrera (1995)	US 1979–1993	Treatment	Heroin	2.5(–)	16(–)
Gossop et al. (2002b)	UK 1995–1999	Treatment	Heroin, amphetamine	–(–)	18(–)
Gronbladh et al. (1990)	Sweden 1967–1988	Treatment, untreated	Heroin	4.4(0)	15(0)
Hser et al. (2001)	US 1962–1997	Treatment	Narcotics	–(–)	40(1)
Joe et al. (1982)	US 1969–1979	Treatment	Opioids	2.6(0)	17(–)
Langendam et al. (2001)	Holland 1985–1996	Treatment/community	Heroin, cocaine	17.9(11.1)	59(37)
Maxwell et al. (2005)	US 1994–2002	Deaths in methadone	Opioids	n/a	62(4)
Marx et al. (1994)	Switzerland 1987–1989	Drug-related deaths	Primarily opioids	n/a	7(–)
McAnulty et al. (1995)	US 1989–1991	Not in treatment	IDU	3.5(0)	33(0)
Miotto et al. (1997)	US time unspecified	Treatment	Heroin	0(0)	0(0)
Musto & Ramos (1981)	US 1918–1973	Treatment	Morphine	7.6(0)	91(0)
O'Doherty & Farrington (1997)	UK 1986–1991	Opioid deaths	Opioids	n/a	7(3)
Oppenheimer et al. (1994)	UK 1969–1991	Treatment	Heroin	6.3(0)	41(0)
Orti et al. (1996)	Spain 1985–1991	Treatment, hospital	Opioids	–(10.8)	–(36)
Oyefesso et al. (1999)	UK 1974–1993	Notified teenage addicts	Opioids	0.1(0)	1(0)
Perucci et al. (1991)	Italy 1980–1988	Treatment	Opioids	3.5(0.5)	49(8)
Quaglio et al. (2001)	Italy 1985–1998	Treatment	IDU	–(–)	39(33)
Rehm et al. (2005)	Switzerland 1994–2000	Treatment	Heroin	6.9(4.8)	65(45)
Robertson et al. (1994)	UK 1982–1993	GP	IDU	–(7.9)	–(40)

(contd.)

Table 5.1. (*contd.*)

Study	Country/period	Sample	Drug	Crude disease mortality rate (AIDS) per 1000[*]	Proportion of deaths due to disease (AIDS)(%)
Rossow (1994)	Norway 1968–1992	Treatment	"Addicts"	8.6(0.5)	36(2)
Sanchez-Carbonell & Seus (2000)	Spain 1985–1995	Treatment	Heroin	23.1(–)	51(–)
Termorshuizen et al. (2005)	Amsterdam 1985–2002	Treatment and community agencies	IDU	13.5(5.5)	(51)
Tunving (1988)	Sweden 1970–1984	Treatment	Opioids, amphetamine	0(0)	0(0)
Tyndall et al. (2001)	Canada 1996–2000	Community	IDU	–(–)	(18)
Vaillant (1973)	US 1952–1970	Treatment, males	Narcotics	1.0(0)	9(0)
Van Ameijden et al. (1999b)	Holland 1985–1995	Treatment and community agencies	IDU	4.7(–)	27(–)
Van Haarstrecht et al. (1996)	Holland 1985–1993	Treatment, sexually transmitted disease patients	IDU	10.1(4.3)	39(17)
Vlahov et al. (2004)	US 1988–2000	New onset IDU	IDU	21.2(12.4)	65(38)
Wahren et al. (1997)	Sweden 1970–1974	Hospitalised for drug dependence	Stimulants, opioids	3.8(–)	24(–)
Watterson et al. (1975)	US 1970–1974	Treatment	Opioids	5.5(–)	23(–)
Webb et al. (2003)	UK 2000	Drug-related deaths	All	n/a	13(–)
Wille (1981)	UK 1969–1979	Treatment	Heroin	3.8(0)	26(0)
Zador & Sunjic (2000)	Australia 1990–1995	Treatment	Heroin	–	24(13)
Zaccarelli et al. (1994)	Italy 1985–1991	Treatment	IDU	15.0(11.3)	65(49)
Zanis & Woody (1998)	US 1993–1994	Methadone	Heroin	11.8(0)	46(0)

[*]Figures in brackets represents AIDS-related mortality.

living with HIV, and that HIV caused almost 3 million deaths (UNAIDS, 2004). Injecting drug use is an important risk factor for the transmission of blood-borne viral infections (BBVI), the most commonly cited of which are HIV and HCV. Injecting drug use is thought to be the primary factor responsible for the spread of HIV in Eastern Europe, Central Asia, and Latin America (UNAIDS, 2004), and accounts for at least 10% of AIDS cases in high income countries (UNAIDS, 2004). According to the latest Global Burden of Disease Estimates the largest individual cause of death for illicit drug users was AIDS (Degenhardt et al., 2004a).

There is good evidence that the incidence of HIV has increased as a result of the sharing of injecting equipment by IDU in developing societies. The connection between illicit drug use and HIV/AIDS largely arises from injection drug use, via drug users sharing contaminated injecting equipment (Beyrer et al., 2003; Garten et al., 2004; Reid & Costigan, 2002; Stimson, 1993). In the USA and parts of Europe, sharing contaminated needles, syringes, and other injecting equipment accounts for 50% of new HIV notifications (National Centre in HIV Epidemiology and Clinical Research, 2003).

The sharing of injecting equipment is, of course, by no means the only way in which IDU may contract HIV (UNAIDS, 2002). Sexual transmission of the virus is a significant factor within the IDU community, as it is in many communities worldwide. In countries where HIV prevalence is relatively high, IDU with a larger number of sexual partners are more likely to be HIV positive (Doherty et al., 2000). Some IDU may also engage in sex work, which may place them at greater risk of contracting HIV from clients, particularly if they are engaging in highly risky sexual behaviours in the course of their work (Bull et al., 2002; Jones et al., 1998; Persaud et al., 1999; Spittal et al., 2003; Tuan et al., 2004). There is some evidence that stimulant injectors may be more likely than injectors of other drugs to engage in sex work (Chiasson et al., 1991; Darke et al., 1995; Edlin et al., 1994).

5.2.1   *Prevalence and rates of AIDS mortality*

The prevalence of HIV among IDU varies considerably worldwide. In some countries, HIV prevalence among this group may be as high as 80% (Aceijas et al., 2004). In contrast, IDU within some countries with relatively established IDU populations, such as Australia, have a very low prevalence of HIV (1–3%) (Aceijas et al., 2004; National Centre in HIV Epidemiology and Clinical Research, 2003). The low HIV infection rate among Australian IDU is thought to reflect Australia's geographic isolation from countries with high prevalence

of HIV infections. Moreover, the early introduction of needle and syringe programmes in Australia appears to have averted an HIV epidemic among IDU and
their sexual contacts (cf. Chapter 8). The HIV epidemic is a highly dynamic
one: recent years have seen increases in HIV transmission among IDU in
Eastern Europe and Central Asia that are thought to represent the fastest spread
of HIV infection yet observed (Rhodes & Simic, 2005). Even within high
prevalence countries, HIV rates may vary considerably, with rates elevated
within certain areas of some large cities (Aceijas et al., 2004).

HIV/AIDS is a major cause of premature deaths among heroin and other
drug injectors in the USA and Europe (cf. Table 5.1). The cohort studies sum-
marised in Table 5.1 show a considerable variation in mortality rates among
cohorts of drug users due to AIDS, which is not surprising given the large differences in HIV prevalence across the countries from which the cohorts were
drawn, and the time periods over which the cohorts were followed up.

AIDS was not diagnosed before 1981. After the early 1980s major cohorts in
the US and Europe had significant, and increasing, rates of mortality due to
AIDS, with crude rates ranging up to around 10 per thousand person-years
(Davoli et al., 1997; Friedman et al., 1996; Sanchez-Carbonell & Seus, 2000). It
is important to note that other countries, such as Australia and the UK, never
saw similar rates of HIV infection and/or mortality. Furthermore, as these
cohort studies were all conducted in developed countries, it is unclear what the
mortality rates may be among IDU in developing countries where the prevalence of HIV is high, and access to treatment for HIV and heroin dependence
is limited.

Since the 1990s, there appear to have been decreases in mortality due to
AIDS among the high prevalence countries noted above (Bargagli et al., 2001;
Gayet-Ageron et al., 2004). This has coincided to some extent with the advent
of highly active antiretroviral therapies (HAART) (cf. Chapter 8).

5.2.2   *Risk factors for HIV transmission and mortality*

The risk of mortality due to injecting illicit drugs increases with increasing frequency and quantity of injecting (Fischer et al., 1997). Drug users who typically inject drugs daily, or near daily, over periods of years are probably at the
greatest risk of contracting BBVIs (Ross et al., 1992). Studies have repeatedly
found that people who inject cocaine, amphetamines, and "speedballs" (heroin
and cocaine injected together) are at higher risk of HIV infection than the other
IDU (Doherty et al., 2000). High frequency injection is common amongst stimulant users, placing them at a higher risk of contracting blood-borne viruses than

opioid users, who typically inject less frequently (Bux et al., 1995; Chaisson et al., 1989; Tyndall et al., 2003).

There is some evidence that mortality rates due to AIDS differ among sub-populations of IDU. For example, in European cohort studies female IDU have higher AIDS mortality rates than their male counterparts (e.g. Bargagli et al., 2001). Conversely, there has been good evidence observed at a population level to suggest that persons receiving HAART for HIV have a reduced risk of mortality due to AIDS-related causes (Gayet-Ageron et al., 2004). This makes sense because HIV-1 viral load is a significant predictor of progression to AIDS and death among those who are HIV positive (Lyles et al., 1999), and HAART reduces HIV-1 viral load.

IDU with HIV/AIDS are also more likely to die from other causes of mortality than those who are not HIV positive (Eskild et al., 1993; Tyndall et al., 2001; Zaccarelli et al., 1994). This is probably for two reasons: because persons with HIV are immune compromised (and therefore more susceptible to other illnesses), and because of the likelihood that HIV positive status is a marker of broader risk taking behaviours. It is not uncommon for persons infected with HIV, for example, to also be infected with HCV (Benhamou et al., 1999; Maier & Wu, 2002; Poynard, 2004). Some studies have shown that among IDU, the co-infection prevalence of HIV and HCV is as high as 90–95% (Poynard, 2004). There is increasing evidence that people infected with HIV have a more rapid course of HCV infection (Borgia et al., 2003). One study found that IDU who were both HIV and HCV positive had increasing rates of hospitalisation due to complications arising from injecting drug use or liver problems, whereas those who were HIV positive only had decreasing rates of these problems (Gebo et al., 2003).

Among persons receiving HIV treatment, the continued use of illicit drugs may pose risks. There is evidence that the effects of methamphetamine may be greater for HIV positive persons receiving HAART (particularly ritonavir) (Halkitis et al., 2001; Urbina & Jones, 2004). This is because ritonavir has greater affinity for certain enzymes than methamphetamine, so blood levels of methamphetamine (if used concomitantly) may be three to ten times greater than among those not taking ritonavir (Pritzker et al., 2002). There has been one Australian case report of an HIV positive man receiving combination antiretroviral therapy (including ritonavir) who died from a methamphetamine overdose following injection of the drug (Hales et al., 2000). There are also case reports of 3,4-methylenedioxymethamphetamine (MDMA) related fatalities occurring in the same manner (Henry & Hill, 1998). These potential risks need to be investigated further, but would suggest that persons receiving treatment for HIV may be at increased of mortality if using illicit psychostimulant drugs.

5.3   HCV

HCV is a BBVI that affects the liver. The discovery of HCV as a cause of non-A/non-B hepatitis in 1989 permitted the development of a diagnostic test. Following the advent of a diagnostic test for HCV, and screening of donated blood, the transmission of HCV through blood transfusions has been almost completely prevented. As a result, the predominant mode of transmission of HCV in most developed countries is through injecting drug use (Limburg, 2004). It has been estimated that around 170 million people have been infected with HCV around the world (Limburg, 2004). Chronic HCV infection has been estimated to occur in 75% of infections, and 3–11% of chronic HCV carriers will develop liver cirrhosis within 20 years (Hepatitis C Virus Projections Working Group, 1998).

Given the larger number of people infected with HCV, and the more protracted complications arising from this infection, the net health and economic cost of HCV transmitted by injecting drug use may be considerably higher than that of HIV (Hepatitis C Virus Projections Working Group, 1998; Wodak & Lurie, 1996). As will be detailed below, the rates of mortality from HCV infection among cohorts of IDU to date have been lower than those of HIV. This may change as IDU who have chronic HCV infections age, and develop liver cirrhosis and end-stage liver disease.

HCV is spread by the shared use of injecting equipment. It is a more robust virus than HIV and thus more easily spread. The base rate of HCV infection among IDU is substantially higher than the base rate of HIV infection. Thus the risk of contracting HCV from any episode of sharing of injecting equipment is much higher than those for HIV (Crofts et al., 1999).

5.3.1   *Prevalence and rates of mortality associated with HCV*

The prevalence of HCV among IDU is much higher than that of HIV around the world. In many western European countries, rates of HCV infection range from 40% to 90% depending upon the subgroup being studied (Limburg, 2004). In Australia, among needle and syringe programme attendees, between 50% and 60% have been infected with HCV (National Centre in HIV Epidemiology and Clinical Research, 2003).

To date, mortality related to HCV has been lower among IDU than mortality related to HIV. In a cohort of HIV positive persons followed up over a 5-year period, 0.6% died of hepatitis compared to 10% who died of AIDS-related illness (Fugelstad et al., 1995). In a cohort of New York IDU followed over 8 years, 9% of deaths were attributed to cirrhosis (although the role of alcohol could not be determined) (Friedman et al., 1996). In a Stockholm cohort, 4% of deaths over an 8-year period were attributed to cirrhosis (a rate of 1.1 per thousand person-years) (Galli & Musicco, 1994). Rates of cirrhosis are likely to be higher among HIV positive persons: one study estimated that liver disease rates were 2.2 per thousand person-years for HIV positive persons compared to 1.1 per thousand person-years for HIV negative persons (Zaccarelli et al., 1994).

5.3.2   *Risk factors for HCV transmission and mortality*

HCV is largely transmitted through blood to blood contact. A number of factors have been associated with the transmission of HCV. Infection with HCV is thought to occur relatively early in many injectors' careers (Budd et al., 2002; Crofts et al., 1993). As noted above for HIV, more frequent injectors, and those injecting psychostimulants, are likely to be at higher risk of contracting HCV. More recently, there has been some evidence suggesting that HCV may also be transmitted through non-injecting routes of drug administration, specifically through the shared use of "crackpipes" (Tortu et al., 2001, 2004).

The rate of HCV transmission in prison is thought to be significantly higher than in the community (Crofts et al., 1995). Rates of HCV infection are elevated in the prison population, and the sharing of injecting equipment and tattoo equipment among IDU in prison is highly prevalent (Dolan et al., 1996). A previous history of imprisonment has been a consistent predictor of HCV positive status among samples of IDU (Broers et al., 1998).

One demographic factor that has been associated with HCV infection is gender. Some studies have reported higher HCV incidence rates among women (Broers et al., 1998; Budd et al., 2002). This may be due to greater sharing of injecting paraphernalia, with women having more sharing partners (Budd et al., 2002). The situation is unclear, however, as not all research has found this gender difference, and other studies have suggested that males might be at higher risk (Crofts et al., 1993).

5.4   Acute infections due to injecting drug use

Infections other than HIV and HCV amongst IDU may also have devastating consequences for both morbidity and mortality. The most prominent of these is endocarditis, an inflammation of the inside lining of the heart chambers and heart valves (endocardium) (Karch, 2002). IDU contract endocarditis through the sharing of infected injecting equipment. Bacterial infection is the most common source of endocarditis, but it can also be caused by fungi. Infection may result in congestive heart failure, arrhythmias, heart valve damage, blood clots, cerebral infarction, intracranial haemorrhage, and brain abscesses (Karch, 2002; Tunkel & Pradhan, 2002). It should be noted that intracranial infections amongst drug injectors may also occur in the absence of infective endocarditis (Tunkel & Pradhan, 2002): in one study staphylococcus was the most frequent infective organism, followed by streptococci (Carrel et al., 1993).

The relative contribution of such infections to mortality among IDU may be lower than others such as HIV and HCV. One Italian cohort study found 1.5% of deaths were due to septic shock, 0.2% due to tetanus, and a further 0.2% due to endocarditis (Galli & Musicco, 1994). Slightly higher rates were found in a London cohort followed up from an earlier time period: 2.4% of deaths among the cohort were accounted for by endocarditis over the 22-year follow-up period (Oppenheimer et al., 1994).

HIV infection and a previous history of endocarditis have been found to be independent predictors of endocarditis among IDU (Spijkerman et al., 1995; Zaccarelli et al., 1994). In one study, women appeared to be at an increased risk for endocarditis (Spijkerman et al., 1995), while another found that the mean age of patients who died was significantly greater than that of those who survived (Baddour et al., 1991).

5.5   Cardiovascular pathology

5.5.1   *Psychostimulant users*

As discussed in detail in Chapter 4, cardiac pathology is a consistent feature of heavy, chronic users of psychostimulants such as cocaine and methamphetamine, with cocaine being particularly cardiotoxic (Darke et al., 2005a; Karch, 2002; Kaye & McKetin, 2005; Lange & Hillis, 2001; Vasica & Tennant, 2002; Wijetunga et al., 2003). This is not surprising given what is known of the effects of these stimulant drugs (Julien, 2001; Karch, 2002). Cocaine and methamphetamine and both increase the release of noradrenaline and dopamine, leading to increases in heart rate, narrowing or spasm of blood vessels, and increased blood pressure (Julien, 2001; Karch, 2002; Kaye & McKetin, 2005). There is some evidence that methamphetamine may also have damaging effects on cells in the heart that are independent of these effects (Kaye & McKetin, 2005).

Although cardiac pathology is common among chronic and heavy stimulant users, the contribution of such pathology to mortality among this group appears to be less marked. A 10-year follow-up of a cohort of drug users attending a drug treatment clinic in Milan estimated that deaths due to myocardial infarction occurred at a rate of 0.2 per thousand person-years (0.7% of all deaths amongst the cohort) (Galli & Musicco, 1994). Among IDU in Rome, the rate of mortality per thousand person-years due to cardiovascular problems was 0.9 among HIV positive persons and 0.2 for HIV negative persons (Zaccarelli et al., 1994). In Stockholm, cardiovascular disease accounted for 2% of deaths among a cohort of drug dependent persons followed for 12 years (Fugelstad et al., 1997). The rate was higher among a cohort of highly disadvantaged drug users followed up for 8 years in New York, where heart disease accounted for 10% of deaths (Friedman et al., 1996).

5.5.2 *Cannabis users*

One of the most consistent effects of cannabis in humans and animals is an increased heart rate, an effect related to the concentration of tetrahydro-cannabinol (THC) in the blood (Hall et al., 2001). Healthy young adults are only mildly stressed by these cardiovascular effects (Tennant, 1983). There is no evidence that these effects permanently damage the cardiovascular system, although patients with cardiovascular problems may not fare so well. Whether this translates into increased mortality risks for those using cannabis may become clearer as cohorts of heavy cannabis users age, and enter the risk period for cardiovascular disease (Hall et al., 2001).

An increase in heart rate is more common among occasional cannabis users than regular users, because regular users become tolerant to effects of THC (Chesher & Hall, 1999; Hall et al., 2001; Rubin & Comitas, 1975; Stefanis et al., 1977). Given that most young adults only occasionally smoke cannabis, and generally cease cannabis use in their late 20s or early 30s, it does not seem likely that cannabis causes heart disease among a large proportion of younger cannabis users (Bachman et al., 1997; Hall et al., 2001). Adverse cardiovascular effects may occur in a minority of users who continue to use cannabis into later adulthood (when the risk for heart disease is highest). A recent study estimated that a 44-year-old adult who used cannabis daily would increase their annual risk of an acute cardiovascular event by 1.5–3% (Mittleman et al., 2001). Given that only 3.5% of all cardiac patients had smoked cannabis in the previous year, and only 0.2% of the patients with myocardial infarction reported cannabis use, the number of myocardial infarctions attributable to the use of cannabis appears to be extremely small. This might change as cohorts of cannabis users age and the prevalence of cannabis use increases among this older age group.

Another recent study found that the use of cannabis in a young adult population was not associated with the presence of calcium in coronary arteries (an indicator of coronary atherosclerosis) (Sidney, 2003). Similarly, a cohort study conducted in a large health maintenance organisation showed no association between cannabis use and admission to hospital for myocardial infarction or coronary heart disease (Sidney, 2002).

5.6   Cancer and cannabis use

Given the widespread use of cannabis worldwide, there is comparatively little research conducted on the relationship between the cancer and cannabis use. Two cohort studies have examined the effects of regular, prolonged cannabis use on risks of cancer (Hall et al., 2001). One of these reported no increase in overall rates among cannabis users (although there were slightly increased rates of prostate and cervical cancer) (Sidney et al., 1997). A second study found twice the odds of aerodigestive cancers among heavy users of cannabis, however, it was difficult to determine the role of cannabis smoking, as distinct from tobacco smoking, in the development of aerodigestive cancers as many cannabis users also smoked tobacco (Andreasson & Allebeck, 1990).

The longer term follow up of cohorts of cannabis users may still show an increased risk of cancers and mortality, if enough cohort members continue to smoke cannabis (Sidney, 2003). The cohorts to date have not followed cannabis smokers into later adult life, so that it might be too early to detect an increased risk of chronic diseases that are potentially associated with the use of cannabis.

The largely infrequent use of cannabis during young adulthood may reflect the illegality of cannabis. We cannot, however, assume that smoking cannabis would continue to have the same small impact on mortality if its use were to increase in prevalence and/or frequency.

5.7   Summary

There are specific disease risks associated with illicit drug use that increase its salience as a cause of premature death. The two most common infections associated with illicit drug use, and injecting drug use in particular, are HIV and HCV. Overall, the prevalence of HCV among illicit drug users worldwide is higher than that of HIV. More frequent injectors, and those injecting psychostimulants, are at a higher risk of contracting HIV and HCV.

There are other, non-infective, disease risks that are associated with illicit drug use. In particular, cardiac pathology is a consistent feature of heavy, chronic use of psychostimulants, most particularly cocaine and amphetamine. While cannabis affects the cardiovascular system, current evidence indicates that it does not seem likely to cause heart disease among large proportions of cannabis users. This might, however, change as cohorts of cannabis users continue to use cannabis into ages, brackets in which heart disease risk is highest. Cannabis may also be associated with an increased risk of cancer. At this stage, however, it is difficult to exclude the role of concomitant tobacco smoking from the effects of cannabis per se.

Key points: Summary of disease and illicit drug use

- In terms of the major diseases, drug injectors are at particular risk of HIV and HCV.
- Injecting drug use is the primary factor in the spread of HIV in Eastern Europe, Central Asia, and Latin America, and in ≥10% of AIDS cases in high income countries.
- HCV is a BBVI that affects the liver, and is spread by the shared use of injecting equipment.
- Chronic HCV infection has been estimated to occur in 75% of infections, and 3–11% of chronic HCV carriers will develop liver cirrhosis within 20 years.
- More frequent injectors, and those injecting psychostimulants, are at higher risk of contracting HIV and HCV.
- The prevalence of HCV among illicit drug users is higher than that of HIV.
- Drug injectors are also exposed to central nervous system (CNS) infections such as endocarditis, although the risk is lower than for HIV and HCV.
- Cardiac pathology is a consistent feature of heavy, chronic psychostimulant use.
- Cannabis affects the cardiovascular system, but does not seem likely to cause heart disease among a large proportion of cannabis users. This might change as cohorts of cannabis users age.
- Two cohort studies have reported increased risk of cancer associated with cannabis use, but it is difficult to exclude the role of concomitant tobacco smoking.

6

Mortality and suicide

6.1   Introduction

Despite its salience as a cause of death amongst illicit drug users, suicide has been a relatively neglected area of research in the drug and alcohol field. This is curious because, as noted previously, it has long been known that there are extremely high levels of depressive disorders amongst this population (Darke & Ross, 2001; Degenhardt et al., 2001; Dinwiddie et al., 1997; Teesson et al., 2005), and suicide is a leading cause of death amongst illicit drug users. Despite its status as a "hidden issue" of the illicit drug field, however, suicide presents a major clinical challenge to those treating drug-dependent users, and needs to be recognised as such. The current chapter examines rates of suicide, methods employed, and risk factors amongst the general population and illicit drug users. Both completed and attempted suicide are examined, representing two aspects of a single phenomenon.

6.2   Suicide amongst the general population

Rates of completed suicide in the general population vary greatly from country to country. For example, rates higher than 0.3 per thousand are reported in Finland, Hungary, and Sri Lanka compared to rates of approximately 0.1 per thousand in the US, UK, and Australia (Diekstra & Gulbinat, 1993; Hassan, 1995; Lynskey et al., 2000). Despite differences in suicide rates, recent years have seen sharp increase rates of completed suicide in Europe, the Americas, Asia, and Australia (Diekstra & Gulbinat, 1993; Hassan, 1995; Lynskey et al., 2000). The increase in suicide rates seen internationally appears mainly attributable to increases in rates amongst younger males (Diekstra & Gulbinat, 1993; Lynskey et al., 2000). Clearly, such a trend is of direct relevance when discussing suicide among illicit drug users, as males represent the majority of this population, and drug use typically commences in the adolescent years (Chen & Kandel, 1995; Degenhardt et al., 2000; Kandel et al., 1992).

No discussion of suicide as a clinical issue can ignore attempted suicide. As is the case with accidental drug overdose, fatalities represent only a fraction of the overall burden of disease. It has been estimated that the incidence of attempted suicide is 10–20 times that of completed suicide (Diekstra & Gulbinat, 1993). Thus, for every completed suicide, there are between 10 and 20 suicide attempts. Apart from the considerable harm and distress associated with suicide attempts, previous suicide attempts are also strong predictors of subsequent attempts (Gibbs et al., 2005; Harris & Barraclough, 1997; Pokorny, 1983). Major community surveys indicate that the lifetime prevalence of attempted suicide in the general population ranges between 3% and 5% (Table 6.1). Furthermore, up to 2% of the general population attempt suicide in a 12-month period. As would be expected, rates of suicidal ideation exceed actual attempts.

6.3 Suicide amongst illicit drug users

While national suicide rates may vary, the relative risk of completed suicide across a range of drugs is significantly higher than that of the general population (Harris & Barraclough, 1997; Wilcox et al., 2004). Opioid dependence, for instance, is associated with a completed suicide risk 14 times that of the general population (Harris & Barraclough, 1997; Wilcox et al., 2004). Increased risk was not restricted to injectable substances: Harris & Barraclough (1997) also reported that cannabis dependence increased suicide risk nearly 4 times. Excess suicide rates also applied to dependence upon licit drugs. Benzodiazepine dependence

Table 6.1. Attempted suicide and suicidal ideation amongst general population samples

Study	Sample	Attempted suicide		Suicidal ideation	
		Lifetime (%)	12 months (%)	Lifetime (%)	12 months (%)
Borges et al. (2000)	USA	4.6	–		
Brosnich & Wittchen (1994)	Germany	4.1	–	14.7	
Cooper-Patrick et al. (1994)	USA				2.6
Madianos et al. (1994)	Greece		2.6		11.3
Pirkis et al. (2000)	Australia	3.6	0.4	16.0	3.4

is associated with a suicide rate more than 45 times that of matched peers, and alcohol dependence 6 times (Harris & Barraclough, 1997). Excess suicide rates associated with licit drugs are of direct relevance to illicit drug users, as there are high rates of use and dependence upon these drugs seen amongst this group (cf. Darke & Ross, 1997a).

The excess risk referred to above indicates that illicit drug users are at substantially greater risk of death through suicide than non-drug users. The impact of this increased risk on illicit drug mortality is demonstrated by the proportion of deaths attributed to suicide (Table 6.2). As would be expected, given the suicide specific standardised mortality ratios (SMRs) reported above, a substantial minority of these deaths result from completed suicide. Table 6.2 presents studies of illicit drug users in which suicide as a cause of death has been reported. It can be seen that in a large proportion of these studies, more than 10% of deaths were attributed to suicide. Table 6.2 clearly indicates the salience of suicide as a clinical issue that impacts substantially upon mortality. Crude suicide rates in longitudinal studies range as high as 7.9 per thousand (Engstrom et al., 1991). In approximately half of longitudinal studies, the crude suicide mortality rate exceeded 2.0 per thousand. It will be recalled that, by comparison, population rates are in the order of 0.1–0.3 per thousand. What is also clear from Table 6.2 is that suicide is a major issue for users across a range of drug classes, and not merely opioids. High levels of death due to suicide are also seen among cocaine and amphetamine users. It is clear that a clinically significant component of the excess mortality that is seen amongst illicit drug users is directly attributable to suicide.

Given the high rates of completed suicide among illicit drug users, it would be expected that the rates of attempted suicide would also be high. In all studies in which attempted suicide has been measured, the prevalence of attempted suicide is many orders of magnitude greater than those reported amongst community samples (Table 6.3). Lifetime histories of attempted suicide range between 17% and 43%, compared to 5% or under amongst community samples. In the majority of studies, more than a third of participants have histories of attempted suicide. The fact that a previous suicide attempt is a strong predictor of a subsequent attempt (Gibbs et al., 2005; Harris & Barraclough, 1997; Pokorny, 1983), illustrates the threat to life, and the extent of the clinical problem facing those who treat illicit drug users.

It is of clinical importance that these attempts are not merely incidents that occurred in the person's distant past. Where recent attempts have been measured, annual rates have ranged between 6% and 13% (Table 6.3). In fact, the annual rate of suicide attempts amongst illicit drug users is higher than the *lifetime* prevalence of the general population.

Table 6.2. Suicide as a cause of death amongst illicit drug users

Study	Country/period	Sample	Drug	Crude suicide rate (per 1000 person-years)	Proportion of deaths due to suicide (%)
Bartu et al. (2004)	Australia 1985–1998	Hospital/psychiatric admissions	Opioids. amphetamine	0.3	19
Benson & Holmberg (1984)	Sweden 1968–1978	Conscripts, rehabilitation and psychiatric patients, welfare recipients	Cannabis, solvents, last stage of delirium (LSD), stimulants	2.9	64
Bentley & Busuttil (1996)	UK 1989–1994	Coronial cases	Opioids	n/a	9
Bewley et al. (1968)	UK 1947–1966	Notified addicts	Heroin	6.2	23
Bucknall & Robertson (1986)	UK 1981–1985	General practitioner (GP) attendees	Heroin	1.4	14
Caplehorn et al. (1996)	Australia 1979–1991	Treatment	Heroin	1.4	12
Darke et al. (2005a)	Australia 1993–2002	Coronial cases	Cocaine	n/a	3
Dukes et al. (1992)	New Zealand 1971–1989	Treatment	Opioids	0.9	12
Engstrom et al. (1991)	Sweden 1973–1984	Drug-related hospitalisation	Amphetamine, cocaine, heroin	7.9	35
Eskild et al. (1993)	Norway 1985–1991	Human immunodeficiency virus (HIV) test centre	IDU	2.4	10
Fugelstad et al. (1995)	Sweden1986–1990	HIV + drug addicts	Heroin	5.0	13

(contd.)

Table 6.2. (*contd.*)

Study	Country/period	Sample	Drug	Crude suicide rate (per 1000 person-years)	Proportion of deaths due to suicide (%)
Fugelstad et al. (1997)	Sweden 1981–1992	Drug-related hospitalisation	Heroin, amphetamine	2.2	14
Galli & Musicco (1994)	Italy 1980–1991	Treatment	Methadone	0.6	2
Gardner (1970)	UK 1965–1969	Coronial cases	Opioids	n/a	14
Gill et al. (2002)	USA 1997–2000	Coronial	MDMA	n/a	0
Goldstein & Herrera (1995)	USA 1979–1993	Treatment	Heroin	0.5	3
Gronbladh et al. (1990)	Sweden 1967–1988	Treatment, untreated	Heroin	0.9	3
Haarstrep & Jepson (1988)	Denmark 1973–1984	Treatment	Opioids	6.1	23
Karch et al. (1999)	USA 1985–1997	Coronial	Amphetamine	n/a	12
Langendam et al. (2001)	Holland 1985–1996	Treatment/community	Heroin, cocaine	2.2	7
Logan et al. (1998)	USA 1993–1995	Coronial	Amphetamine	n/a	21
Maxwell et al. (2005)	USA 1994–2002	Deaths in methadone	Opioids	n/a	5
Marx et al. (1994)	Switzerland 1987–1989	Drug-related deaths	Primarily opioids	n/a	6
Miotto et al. (1997)	USA time unspecified	Treatment	Heroin	–	25
Musto & Ramos (1981)	USA	Treatment	Morphine	0.2	2
O'Doherty & Farrington (1997)	UK 1986–1991	Opioid deaths	Opioids	n/a	3

Study	Location/period	Sample	Drug		
Oppenheimer et al. (1994)	UK 1969–1991	Treatment	Heroin	0.7	5
Oyefesso et al. (1999b)	UK 1974–1993	Notified teenage addicts	Opioids	0.1	3
Perucci et al. (1991)	Italy 1980–1988	Treatment	Opioids	0.3	5
Quaglio et al. (2001)	Italy 1985–1998	Treatment	IDU	–	6
Raikos et al. (2002)	Greece 1998–2000	Coronial	MDMA	n/a	0
Rehm et al. (2005)	Switzerland 1994–2005	Treatment	Heroin	1.7	16
Rossow (1994)	Norway 1968–1992	Treatment	"Addicts"	3.5	15
Shaw (1999)	Taiwan 1991–1996	Coronial	Amphetamine	n/a	11
Tunving (1988)	Sweden 1970–1984	Treatment	Opioids, amphetamine	3.3	31
Vaillant (1973)	USA 1952–1970	Treatment, males	Narcotics	2.0	17 (suicide/homicide)
Van Ameijden et al. (1999a)	Holland 1985–1995	Treatment and community agencies	IDU	5.9	34
Van Haarstrecht et al. (1996)	Holland 1985–1993	Treatment, sexually transmitted disease (STD) patients	IDU	3.6	21
Wahren et al. (1997)	Sweden 1971–1990	Hospitalised for drug dependence	Stimulants, opioids	3.0	19
Wille (1981)	UK 1969–1979	Treatment	Heroin	0.8	5
Zador & Sunjic (2000)	Australia 1990–1995	Treatment	Heroin	–	8
Zaccarelli et al. (1994)	Italy 1985–1991	Treatment	IDU	0.4	2
Zanis & Woody (1998)	USA 1993–1994	Methadone	Heroin	0	0
Zhu et al. (2000)	Japan 1994–1998	Coronial	Amphetamine	n/a	0

Table 6.3. Attempted suicide and suicidal ideation amongst illicit drug users

Study	Sample	Attempted suicide		Suicidal ideation	
		Lifetime (%)	12 months (%)	Lifetime (%)	12 months (%)
Allison et al. (1985)	USA, Methadone entrants	–	6	–	23
Darke et al. (2001)	Australia, Methadone patients	40	10	–	24
Darke et al. (2004)	Australia, heroin treatment entrants	34	13	–	23
Darke et al. (2005e)	Australia, heroin treatment	32	9	–	7
Darke & Kaye (2004)	Australia, cocaine users	28	7	–	–
Dinwiddie et al. (1992)	USA, mixed IDU	24	–	–	–
Johnsson & Fridell (1997)	Sweden, treatment entrants	45	–	–	–
Gossop et al. (1998)	UK, treatment entrants	–	–	–	29
Kosten & Rounsaville (1988)	USA, treatment entrants	17	5.5*	–	21*
Lynskey et al. (2004)	USA, cannabis users	13	–	51	–
Murphy et al. (1983)	USA, entering/in treatment	17	–	–	–
Ravndal & Vaglum (1999)	Norway, treatment entrants	47	27**	–	–
Rossow & Lauritzen (1999)	Norway, treatment entrants	33	–	–	–
Rossow & Lauritzen (2001)	Norway, treatment entrants	38	–	–	42#
Roy (2001)	USA, cocaine treatment patients	39	–	–	–
Roy (2002)	USA, heroin treatment patients	43	–	–	–
Vingoe et al. (1999)	UK, in treatment	35	8	60	55

*2.5 years; **5years; #month.

Whilst the majority of the samples listed are primarily composed of opioid users, two studies have specifically examined attempted suicide amongst cocaine users (Darke & Kaye, 2004; Roy, 2001). In both studies, rates of attempted suicide were comparable to those reported among opiate users. Importantly, suicide attempts are not restricted to injecting drug users (IDUs). Darke & Kaye (2004) reported that 10% of cocaine users who had never injected a drug also had such histories. Similarly, 13% of cannabis users in Lynskey et al. (2004) had made at least one suicide attempt.

As would be expected from the high rates of completed and attempted suicide, the prevalence of suicidal ideation among illicit drug users is also far in excess of community samples (Table 6.3). Suicidal ideation is, not surprisingly, a strong predictor of a future suicide attempt (Beck et al., 1985; Pirkis et al., 2000). A recent study found that 12% of those reporting suicidal ideation went on to make an attempt within 12 months (Pirkis et al., 2000). More specifically, heroin users who report suicidal ideation are also highly likely to make an attempt within 12 months (Darke et al., 2005e).

6.4   Methods of suicide

The means by which illicit drug users attempt or complete suicide is of clinical relevance, both for suicide prevention and our understanding of the relationship between overdose and suicide. While amongst the general population the most common methods for suicide are poisoning, hanging, and gunshot wounds, important gender differences exist (Beautrais et al., 1996; Canetto & Sakinofsky, 1998; Denning et al., 2001; Hassan, 1995; Rich et al., 1988). Males predominantly employ violent methods for suicide, such as shooting, and hanging. In contrast, females are more likely to employ non-violent methods, such as poisoning or carbon monoxide. The fact that males predominantly employ violent methods, and females non-violent methods may well explain the predominance of males in completed suicides, and of females amongst suicide attempts, as violent methods clearly are more likely to cause death. Poisoning with drugs constitutes only a small minority of male fatalities in the general population, but represents half of female cases.

To date, few studies have reported on the methods of suicide employed by illicit drug users (Bucknall & Robertson, 1986; Darke & Kaye, 2004; Darke et al., 2001; Dukes et al., 1992; Engstrom et al., 1991; Gardner, 1970; Johnsson & Fridell, 1997; Marx et al., 1994; Oyefesso et al., 1999a, b; Rossow, 1994; Tunving, 1988; Vingoe et al., 1999). When examining the methods of suicide used by illicit drug users it needs to be borne in mind that, as amongst the general population, illicit drug users who complete suicide are predominantly male (e.g. Dukes et al., 1992; Goldstein & Herrera, 1995; Perucci et al., 1991; Quaglio et al., 2001; Rossow, 1994). Similarly, those who attempt suicide are predominantly female (e.g. Borges et al., 2000; Darke & Kaye, 2004; Darke et al., 2005e; Johnsson & Fridell, 1997; Ravndal & Vaglum, 1999; Rossow & Lauritzen, 2001; Roy, 2001, 2002). Unfortunately, however, the studies that have examined methods of suicide amongst illicit drug users rarely report gender-specific data. Studies reporting methods employed in cases of fatal suicide among illicit drug users show substantially higher proportions of substance poisoning deaths than would be expected amongst a general population sample (Bucknall & Robertson, 1986; Dukes et al., 1992; Engstrom et al., 1991; Gardner, 1970; Marx et al., 1994; Oyefesso et al., 1999a, b; Rossow, 1994; Tunving, 1988). Overall, drug overdose as a means of suicide appears to occur in approximately a half or more of cases. By way of comparison, only 17% of completed suicides in New York were attributed to drug poisoning (Denning et al., 2001). Thus, whilst males constitute the bulk of illicit drug user suicide cases, poisoning still dominates amongst this population. As in the broader population, violent deaths are common among illicit drug user suicides, but do not appear to occur at the rate seen in non-drug users.

Similar patterns to those seen in completed suicides amongst illicit drug users are reported for attempted suicide (Darke & Kaye, 2004; Darke et al., 2001; Johnsson & Fridell, 1997; Vingoe et al., 1999). Thus, drug poisoning has dominated suicide attempts amongst samples of opioid (Darke et al., 2001; Vingoe et al., 1999), cocaine (Darke & Kaye, 2004), and mixed illicit drug users (Johnsson & Fridell, 1997). Given that females represent the majority of suicide attempts amongst illicit drug users, the predominance of poisoning might be expected. Overall, however, the use of drugs in completed or attempted suicide appears to be over-represented among illicit drug users.

It is perhaps not surprising that there is an excess of drug poisoning deaths amongst illicit drug users. By definition, these groups have access to, and use, drugs. What is interesting, however, are the relatively low proportions of cases attributed to overdose from the primary drug of dependence. Rather, the substances most implicated are *licit* pharmaceuticals, primarily benzodiazepines, and antidepressants (Bucknall & Robertson, 1986; Darke & Kaye, 2004; Darke et al., 1992, 2001; Johnsson & Fridell, 1997; Rossow, 1994; Tunving, 1988; Vingoe et al., 1999). The use of these drugs is extremely common amongst illicit drug users (Darke & Ross, 2000a; Gossop et al., 2001; Kidorf et al., 1996; Ross et al., 1996). Thus, whilst drug overdose is a leading means of completed and attempted suicide amongst drug users, it is non-opioid prescription pharmaceuticals that constitute the bulk of cases. Such findings have direct implications for the attribution of intentionality to death due to drug overdose.

The most intriguing example of this phenomenon relates to heroin. As discussed in detail elsewhere, heroin is a drug that results in substantial numbers of overdoses, both fatal and non-fatal. Despite this, and the obvious toxicity of the drug, deliberate heroin overdose does not appear to be the suicide method of choice among heroin users. The relationship between heroin overdose and suicide, however, will always be problematic due to ambiguous circumstantial information, high levels of clinical depression, and unclear intent (Cantor et al., 2001). A statistical association between heroin overdose and suicide has been noted (Best et al., 2000; Murphy et al., 1983; Neale, 2000; Rossow & Lauritzen, 1999; Vingoe et al., 1999), and it has been argued that suicidal intent is present in a large proportion of overdose cases (Best et al., 2000; Neale, 2000). Other studies, however, cast doubt upon this relationship (Darke & Ross, 2001; Darke et al., 2000; Johnsson & Fridell, 1997; Kosten & Rounsaville, 1988; Ravndal & Vaglum, 1999; Rossow, 1994). Recent studies of heroin- and cocaine-related fatalities (Darke et al., 2000, 2004) reported that 5% and 8% of cases respectively were deliberate overdoses. Even if these figures are regarded as conservative, deliberate overdose appears unusual. Conversely, if one examines suicide among heroin users, deliberate overdoses constitute only a small proportion of completed and attempted suicides (Bucknall & Robertson, 1986; Darke & Ross, 2001; Darke et al., 2000; Dukes et al., 1992; Johnsson & Fridell, 1997; Rossow, 1994; Tunving, 1988; Vingoe et al., 1999). Whilst it must be accepted that there are problems differentiating deliberate and accidental overdose, the overall pattern appears to indicate that most overdoses are accidental, and most illicit drug user suicides employ means other than their drug of dependence. Why this should be the case is intriguing. Drug users have access to their drug of choice, and in the case of opioids this is an obvious means of self-poisoning. It is possible that drug users associate their drug with pleasure, rather than a means of suicide.

6.5   Risk factors

Apart from substance dependence, risk factors for suicide fall into four broad areas: demographic characteristics, psychopathology, family dysfunction, and social isolation/dysfunction (Table 6.4). With the exception of gender, the risk factors for both attempted and completed suicide are essentially the same (Beautrais et al., 1996; Pokorny, 1983). These factors increase the risk of an attempt on the person's life, regardless of the outcome of that behaviour.

Table 6.4. Major risk factors for suicide

Risk factor	Comment
Gender	
Completed suicide	Males 3 times more likely
Attempted suicide	Females 3 times more likely
Age	Younger at greater risk. Age risk corresponds with peak drug using ages
Psychopathology	
Major depression/dysthymia	Major risk factor
Anxiety disorders	Increased risk
Borderline personality disorder	Strong association with suicide
Conduct disorder	Increased risk
Antisocial personality disorder	Risk equivocal, highly over-diagnosed
Post-traumatic stress disorder	Increased risk
Family dysfunction	
Parental separation prior to age 15	Increased risk
Family social disadvantage	Increased risk for low socio-economic groups
Parental psychopathology	Increased risk (parental mood disorders, suicide)
Childhood sexual abuse	Increased risk
Childhood physical abuse	Increased risk
Social isolation/disadvantage	
Lack of social support	Socially isolated at greater risk
Unemployment	Increased risk
Homelessness	Increased risk
Drug use	
Use of illicit substances	Increased risk
Polydrug use	Greater risk with more extensive polydrug use

One of the outstanding features of the risk factors presented in Table 6.4 is that they are almost a re-description of the illicit drug-dependent population. In particular, regular, dependent users of opioids, cocaine, and amphetamine all have an extremely high prevalence of these risk factors when compared to the general population. All of these factors, with the exception of antisocial personality disorder (ASPD), have been associated with increased suicide risk among drug users (Darke & Ross, 2001; Johnsson & Fridell, 1997; Rossow & Lauritzen, 2001). Given their widespread exposure to multiple suicide risk factors, it is not surprising that the rates of both completed and attempted suicide amongst illicit drug users are many times greater than those observed amongst the general community.

6.5.1 Demographics

A gender imbalance amongst both attempted and completed suicides is a consistent feature of the literature on suicide (Diekstra & Gulbinat, 1993; Hassan, 1995; Lynskey et al., 2000). Overall, females are greatly over-represented among suicide attempts, being three times more likely than males to make an attempt. In contrast, males form the bulk of completed suicide cases, and are three times more likely to complete suicide. The fact that males are more likely to employ violent methods of suicide, with a higher likelihood of death, may account for this discrepancy. As noted above, illicit drug users reflect this broader population pattern.

Suicide is particularly prevalent amongst the young, with suicide rates being highest amongst teenagers and those aged in their 20s (Diekstra & Gulbinat, 1993; Hassan, 1995; Lynskey et al., 2000; Pokorny, 1983). These ages broadly correspond to those in which the rates of illicit drug use are highest (Chen & Kandel, 1995; Degenhardt et al., 2000; Kandel et al., 1992). Thus, apart from other risk factors, illicit drug users broadly lay in the age range in which suicide behaviours are frequent. It should be noted that there is a second demographic peak in suicide amongst the elderly which is not, however, of direct relevance to the population under discussion.

6.5.2 Psychopathology

A range of psychopathology has been associated with suicidal behaviours. Not surprisingly, mood disorders have a particularly strong relationship to suicide. Major depression is strongly related to both attempted and completed suicide (Harris & Barraclough, 1997; Hassan, 1995; Pokorny, 1983). Specifically, major depression has been estimated to increase the risk of completed suicide by a factor of 20. Dysthymia, a less severe mood disorder than clinical depression, is associated with a 12-fold increase in risk of completed suicide (Harris & Barraclough, 1997). Levels of depressive mood disorders amongst illicit drug using populations are many orders of magnitude greater than those seen amongst non-drug users (Darke & Ross, 2001; Degenhardt et al., 2001; Dinwiddie et al., 1997; Teesson et al., 2005), and have been specifically related to suicidal behaviours in these populations (Darke et al., 2005e).

Anxiety disorders, including panic disorders and agoraphobia, have been associated a 6–12 times increased risk of completed suicide (Harris & Barraclough, 1997). In particular, the diagnosis of post-traumatic stress disorder (PTSD) is strongly associated with suicide (American Psychiatric Association, 2000). PTSD is an anxiety disorder resulting from traumatic exposure to life-threatening events. As will be discussed more fully later (Chapter 7), dependent illicit drug users repeatedly demonstrate extremely high rates of traumatic exposure and of PTSD when compared to the general population (Mills et al., 2005), and the diagnosis has been related specifically to suicidal behaviours amongst illicit drug users (Darke et al., 2005e; Mills et al., 2005).

Personality disorders, as a group, have been related to attempted suicide and, are associated with a 7-fold increased risk of completed suicide (Harris & Barraclough, 1997). Rates of personality disorder are extremely high in illicit drug using samples, particularly ASPD and Borderline Personality Disorder (BPD). The latter is of particular interest, as approximately 10% of those diagnosed with BPD die by suicide (American Psychiatric Association, 2000). As noted, rates of BPD are high among illicit drug users, and the diagnosis has been specifically related to suicidal behaviours amongst these populations (Darke et al., 2004, 2005d, e; Trull et al., 2000).

Childhood conduct disorder is a diagnosis associated with substantially elevated risk of subsequent attempted and completed suicide (Fergusson & Lynskey, 1995; Shaffer et al., 1996). The diagnosis has also been specifically related to attempted suicide amongst opiate users (Darke et al., 2003c). The evidence associating the adult equivalent of this diagnosis, ASPD, with suicide is equivocal (Beautrais et al., 1996; Casey, 1989; Darke & Ross, 2001; Kjelsberg et al., 1995; Miles, 1977). More specifically, studies have repeatedly failed to find such an association amongst drug users (Buckstein et al., 1993; Darke & Ross, 2001; Darke et al., 2004, 2005e; Dinwiddie et al., 1992; Kjelsberg et al., 1995; Murphy et al., 1983). There are, however, major problems with over-diagnosis of ASPD when used in relation to drug users (Darke et al., 1998). The diagnosis of ASPD primarily focuses on criminal behaviours (American Psychiatric Association, 2000). The criminal behaviours engendered by illicit drug dependence thus means that the odds of receiving a diagnosis ASPD are high. As such, many ASPD diagnoses in this group are artefacts of illicit drug use per se, rather than true diagnoses of psychopathy (Darke et al., 1998).

Overall, it would appear that it is mood disorders, anxiety disorders (particularly PTSD), and BPD that are of the greatest clinical concern for increased suicide risk among illicit drug users.

6.5.3   *Family dysfunction*

A history of family dysfunction or disadvantage strongly predicts suicidal behaviours (Fergusson & Lysnkey, 1995; Hassan, 1995; Spirito et al., 1989).

In particular, low socio-economic status, parental separation prior to age 15, and parental psychopathology (particularly depression) have all been associated with suicidal behaviours. It is also known that a history of either childhood sexual or physical abuse substantially increases risk of suicide (Beautrais et al., 1996; Garnefski & Diekstra, 1997).

Like suicide, illicit drug dependence is strongly associated with family dysfunction, including high rates of parental alcoholism, parental psychopathology, and parental divorce (Darke & Ross, 2001; Johnsson & Fridell, 1997; Rossow & Lauritzen, 1999, 2001). Drug-dependent individuals, and female drug users in particular, also have high levels of childhood physical and sexual abuse (Medrano et al., 1999).

The risk factors described above have been specifically related to illicit drug using populations. Thus, elevated rates of parental psychopathology, absence of parents during childhood, parental substance abuse problems, a history of psychiatric treatment in childhood, and childhood sexual/physical abuse have been strongly related to subsequent attempted or completed suicide amongst illicit drug users (Buckstein et al., 1993; Chatham et al., 1995; Darke & Ross, 2001; Johnsson & Fridell, 1997; Murphy et al., 1983; Rossow & Lauritzen, 2001). The more childhood problems per se illicit drug users have experienced the greater the likelihood of attempted suicide (Rossow & Lauritzen, 2001).

6.5.4 Social isolation

Not surprisingly, social isolation and disadvantage increase the risk of suicide (Appleby et al., 1999; Hassan, 1995; Pokorny, 1983). In particular, perceived lack of social support, unemployment, and homelessness all heighten the risk of suicidal behaviours (Appleby et al., 1999; Hassan, 1995; Pokorny, 1983). What is of direct clinical relevance here is that this picture is almost a re-description of those heavily dependent on heroin, amphetamine, and cocaine, although not typical of recreational methylenedioxymethamphetamine (MDMA) users. The social profile of heavily dependent illicit drug users has repeatedly been shown to be one of predominant unemployment, low educational levels, homelessness, social isolation, and repeated incarceration (Darke & Ross, 2001; Johnson & Fridell, 1997; Rossow & Lauritzen, 1999, 2001). More particularly, social isolation and dysfunction have been specifically related to attempted suicide among illicit drug users (Borges et al., 2000; Chatham et al., 1995; Darke & Ross, 2001; Kosten & Rounsaville, 1988; Rossow & Lauritzen, 1999).

Incarceration is an aspect of social isolation that is particularly prominent amongst illicit drug users. It is not unusual, for instance, to find that half of

IDUs have been imprisoned, and arrests and impending imprisonment have been related to attempted suicide (Buckstein et al., 1993; Darke & Ross, 2001; Joe et al., 1982; Marx et al., 1994). Imprisonment is a consequence of illicit drug user that provides an elevated risk of suicide over that of the general population.

6.5.5 Drug use

In addition to general suicide risk factors, illicit drug users appear to be exposed to risk through their drug use, in that the use of illicit drugs per se is associated with higher risk of attempted suicide (Borges et al., 2000; Lynskey et al., 2005; Petronis et al., 1990). Data from the US National Comorbidity Survey reported increased risk of suicide amongst users of heroin, cocaine, amphetamine, hallucinogens, cannabis, and inhalants (Borges et al., 2000). Heroin dependence, as opposed to use per se, further increased suicide risk, which was not the case for cocaine, amphetamines, or cannabis (Borges et al., 2000).

One of the most important findings to emerge from the Borges et al. (2000) study was that the extent of polydrug use was a stronger predictor of suicidal behaviour than the use of any individual drug class. This is of particular concern for, as has been repeatedly emphasised, extensive polydrug use is the norm among illicit drug using populations. More particularly, extensive polydrug use has been associated with attempted suicide amongst heroin, cocaine, and amphetamine users (Borges et al., 2000; Darke & Ross, 2001; Darke & Kaye, 2004; Darke et al., 2004, 2005e; Murphy et al., 1983; Rossow & Lauritzen, 1999). Thus, even within a group of polydrug users, more extensive use further increases suicide risk. It is important to note that the polydrug use of illicit drug users is by no means restricted to illicit substances. In particular, large proportions also meet criteria for alcohol and/or benzodiazepine dependence and, as discussed previously, both of these are associated with an increased risk of suicide in and of themselves.

Why does polydrug use increase risk, even amongst those already at great risk? One possible reason is that polydrug use reflects severity of distress. Thus, the more extensive polydrug user is under greater psychological distress, and the polydrug use is an attempt at self-medication. Consistent with this hypothesis, more extensive polydrug dependence has been associated with more extensive psychopathology amongst IDUs (Darke & Ross, 1997). Alternatively, it is possible that increased suicide risk may relate to the direct psychological effects of the different drugs themselves. These two theories are not, of course, antithetical, and may reinforce each other.

6.6 Summary of mortality and suicide

Suicide is a major cause of death amongst illicit drug users, and represents a major clinical challenge to those treating people with substance-dependence problems. Overall, what distinguishes groups of dependent illicit drug users from the broader population is the overwhelming range of risk factors that they present with. Indeed, the risk factors for suicide are almost a re-description of the drug-dependent population. In addition, polydrug-use patterns themselves represent additional risk not seen in non-drug using populations. The use of the primary drug of choice to commit suicide, however, appears uncommon. Overdose and suicide should be seen as distinct clinical issues amongst drug users, that requires different clinical responses. As noted at the beginning of this chapter, suicide amongst illicit drug users has been a neglected field. In Chapters 8 and 9 means of reducing suicide rates amongst illicit drug users, and suggested research priorities are discussed.

Key points: Summary of suicide and illicit drug use

- Rates of completed and attempted suicide amongst illicit drug users are many magnitudes higher than those seen amongst the general population.
- In the majority of studies, 10% or more of illicit drug users died by suicide.
- Poisoning by pharmaceuticals is the most common method employed for suicide by drug users, and is more common than amongst the general population.
- Deliberate overdose by the primary drug of dependence appears uncommon.
- Illicit drug users have substantially higher rates of suicide risk factors than the general population, including psychopathology, family dysfunction, social isolation and social dysfunction.
- Polydrug use represents an additional risk factor for illicit drug users over and above those shared with non-drug users.

7

Mortality and trauma

7.1 Introduction

In this chapter we examine deaths attributable to trauma. Death from trauma among illicit drug users is understudied by comparison with overdose and human immunodeficiency virus (HIV)/acquired immunodeficiency syndrome (AIDS), but, nonetheless, there are strong reasons for believing that it plays a role in premature mortality. Firstly, there are lifestyle factors surrounding illicit drug use that suggest that trauma may play a significant role in causing illicit drug user deaths. Illicit drugs are expensive, and highly sought after by dependent drug users. The scope for violence in such circumstances is high. High levels of crime and sex work performed to support drug use are well documented (Flynn et al., 2003; Gossop et al., 1998; Kaye et al., 1998), activities that carry a high trauma risk. At the psychological level, there is a strong association between antisocial personality disorder (ASPD), borderline personality disorder (BPD) and dependent drug use, diagnoses specifically associated with impulsivity, risk-taking and violent behaviours (American Psychiatric Association, 2000). In addition to the more direct results of the illicit drug using lifestyle, there is also a strong association between motor vehicle accident (MVA) trauma, other accidents and illicit drug use (Kelly et al., 2004; Turk & Tsokos, 2004). Finally, there are the specific psychotropic effects of particular drugs to consider. In particular, psychostimulants, such as cocaine and amphetamine, are associated with paranoia, agitated delirium, and acts of violence (American Psychiatric Association, 2000).

The above factors suggest trauma risk, and rates of traumatic death, may be higher amongst illicit drug users than the general population. The current chapter examines rates of trauma and traumatic death amongst illicit drug users, the nature of such trauma, and associated demographic characteristics. Suicide was dealt with separately in Chapter 6, and does not fall under the rubric of trauma for the purposes of this chapter.

7.2 Prevalence and rates of trauma

Rates of post-traumatic stress disorder (PTSD) are significantly higher amongst illicit drug users than non-drug users (Clark et al., 2001; Cottler et al., 1992; Hien et al., 2000; Mills et al., 2005). PTSD is an anxiety disorder that may develop after having experienced, or witnessed, an event involving actual (or threatened) serious injury or death (American Psychiatric Association, 2000). In particular, cocaine and opioid users appear at greater risk of PTSD. Cottler et al. (1992) reported rates of PTSD amongst opiate and cocaine users significantly higher than those seen amongst cannabis users, hallucinogen users, heavy alcohol users, and non-drug using controls. Levels of PTSD were no higher amongst cannabis users, hallucinogen users, heavy alcohol users than non-drug using controls. In all probability this reflects the high levels of dependence associated with both heroin and cocaine use. The population rate of lifetime PTSD is estimated to be in the order of 7% (Kessler et al., 1995; Norris, 1992). By comparison, reported rates of PTSD amongst opioid users are many orders of magnitude higher than population estimates: 20% (current diagnosis) (Hien et al., 2000), 21% (lifetime diagnosis) (Milby et al., 1996), 29% (lifetime) (Clark et al., 2001), 41% (lifetime) (Mills et al., 2005).

As would be expected from the rates of PTSD, life-threatening events, and serious physical assault in particular, appears to be extremely common amongst opioid users. Reported rates of serious assault during adulthood are extremely high: 34% (Cottler et al., 1992), 43% (Clark et al., 2001), 52% (Hien et al. 2000), and 56% (Mills et al., 2005). By comparison, only 14% of non-drug using controls in Cottler et al. (1992) had been assaulted, as had 15% of participants in a large scale general population survey (Norris, 1992). As was the case with PTSD, Cottler et al. (1992) found significantly higher rates of physical assault amongst opioid/cocaine users than among non-drug users or users of other drugs. Looking more broadly, Mills et al. (2005) reported that half of heroin users had been involved in at least one serious, life-threatening accident. It is clear that, at least amongst dependent opioid and cocaine users, traumatic risk to life is a common occurrence.

The above data clearly show traumatic injury and PTSD are strongly associated with the use of opioids and cocaine. Given these levels of exposure, it would be expected that death due to trauma would constitute a significant proportion of illicit drug user deaths, particularly amongst opiate and cocaine users. This appears to be the case. The proportion of deaths in cohort and coronial studies attributable to trauma has ranged up to 46% (Table 7.1). In half of these studies traumatic injury accounted for more than 10% of deaths. Crude mortality

Table 7.1. Trauma as a cause of death amongst illicit drug users

Study	Country/period	Sample	Drug	Crude trauma mortality rate (per 1000 person years)	Proportion of deaths due to trauma (%)
Bartu et al. (2004)	Australia 1985–1998	Hospital/psychiatric admissions	Opioids, amphetamine	0.1	6
Benson & Holmberg (1984)	Sweden 1968–1978	Conscripts, rehabilitation and psychiatric patients, welfare recipients	Cannabis, solvents, lysergic acid diethylamine (LSD), stimulants	1.5	34
Bentley & Busuttil (1996)	UK 1989–1994	Coronial cases	Opioids	n/a	7
Bewley et al. (1968)	UK 1947–1966	Notified addicts	Heroin	2.4	9
Bucknall & Robertson (1986)	UK 1981–1985	General practitioner attendees	Heroin	1.4	14
Caplehorn et al. (1996)	Australia 1979–1991	Treatment	Heroin	2.3	19
Cherubin et al. (1972)	USA 1964–1968	Notified addicts	Heroin	–	7
Cooncool et al. (1979)	USA 1969–1976	Treatment	Heroin	2.6	46
Davoli et al. (1997)	Italy 1980–1992	Treatment	IDU	2.5	10
Darke et al. (2005a)	Australia 1993–2002	Coronial cases	Cocaine	n/a	3
Dukes et al. (1992)	New Zealand 1971–1989	Treatment	Opioids	1.0	13
Engstrom et al. (1991)	Sweden 1973–1984	Drug-related hospitalisation	Amphetamine, cocaine, heroin	6.4	28
Eskild et al. (1993)	Norway 1985–1991	HIV test centre	IDU	2.2	9
Friedman et al. (1996)	USA 1984–1992	Welfare recipients	Drugs and alcohol	0.6	2
Fugelstad et al. (1995)	Sweden1986–1990	HIV + drug addicts	Heroin	1.1	3

Reference	Country/years	Type	Drug		
Fugelstad et al. (1997)	Sweden 1981–1992	Drug-related hospitalisation	Heroin, amphetamine	2.1	13
Galli & Musicco (1994)	Italy 1980–1991	Treatment	Methadone	1.5	5
Gardner (1970)	UK 1965–1969	Coronial cases	Opioids	n/a	10
Gill et al. (2002)	USA 1997–2000	Coronial	3,4-methylene-dioxymetham-phetamine (MDMA)	n/a	32
Goedert et al. (1995)	Italy 1980–1990	Treatment	Heroin	2.2	14
Goldstein & Herrera (1995)	USA 1979–1993	Treatment	Heroin	2.7	17
Gossop et al. (2002b)	UK 1995–1999	Treatment	Heroin, amphetamine	–	14
Gronbladh et al. (1990)	Sweden 1967–1988	Treatment, untreated	Heroin	0.6	2
Joe et al. (1982)	USA 1969–1979	Treatment	Opioids	3.8	25
Joe & Simpson (1987)	USA 1978–1984	Treatment	Opioids	4.5	29
Karch et al. (1999)	USA 1985–1997	Coronial	Amphetamine	n/a	20
Langendam et al. (2001)	Holland, 1985–1996	Treatment/community	Heroin, cocaine	2.7	9
Logan et al. (1998)	USA 1993–1995	Coronial	Amphetamine	n/a	71
Maxwell et al. (2005)	USA 1994–2002	Deaths in methadone	Opioids	n/a	11
McAnulty et al. (1995)	USA 1989–1991	Not in treatment	IDU	1.6	15
Miotto et al. (1997)	USA 12 months	Treatment	Heroin	0	0
Musto & Ramos (1981)	USA 1918–1973	Treatment	Morphine	0.8	10
O'Doherty & Farrington (1997)	UK 1986–1991	Opioid deaths	Opioids	n/a	13
Oppenheimer et al. (1994)	UK 1969–1991	Treatment	Heroin	1.4	9
Orti et al. (1996)	Spain	Treatment, hospital	Opioids	3.7	12
Oyefesso et al. (1999b)	UK 1974–1993	Notified teenage addicts	Opioids	n/a	3

(contd.)

Table 7.1. (*contd.*)

Study	Country/period	Sample	Drug	Crude trauma mortality rate per 1000 (person-years)	Proportion of deaths due to trauma (%)
Perucci et al. (1991)	Italy 1980–1988	Treatment	Opioids	1.5	21
Quaglio et al. (2001)	Italy 1985–1998	Treatment	IDU	–	11
Rehm et al. (2005)	Switzerland 1994–2000	Treatment	Heroin	0.8	8
Raikos et al. (2002)	Greece 1998–2000	Coronial	MDMA	n/a	86
Tunving (1988)	Sweden 1970–1984	Treatment	Opioids, amphetamine	1.5	13
Vaillant (1973)	USA 1952–1970	Treatment, males	Narcotics	1.0	9
Van Ameijden et al. (1999a)	Holland 1985–1995	Treatment and community agencies	IDU	2.5	14
Van Haarstrecht et al. (1996)	Holland 1985–1993	Treatment, sexually transmitted disease patients	IDU	2.2	7
Vlahov et al. (2004)	USA 1988–2000	New onset IDU	IDU	3.3	10
Wahren et al. (1997)	Sweden	Hospitalised for drug dependence	Stimulants, opioids	2.2	14
Webb et al. (2003)	UK 2000	Drug-related deaths	All	n/a	3
Wille (1981)	UK 1969–1979	Treatment	Heroin	1.6	11
Zador & Sunjic (2000)	Australia 1990–1995	Treatment	Heroin	n/a	17
Zaccarelli et al. (1994)	Italy 1985–1991	Treatment	IDU	2.0	9
Zanis & Woody (1998)	USA 1993–1994	Methadone	Heroin	0	0
Zhu et al. (2000)	Japan 1994–1998	Coronial	Amphetamine	n/a	53

rates in most cohort studies were in excess of 2.0 per thousand person-years (Table 7.1).

How do these mortality rates compare to those of the general population? The population mortality rate due to accidents is approximately 0.04 per thousand (Australian Bureau of Statistics, 2004; Centers for Disease Control, 2003; Office of National Statistics, 2004). In almost all cohort studies presented in Table 7.1, rates far exceed these levels. Few studies have directly compared trauma-specific mortality rates of drug users with the general population. Consistent with the high crude mortality rates, these studies have reported substantial excess trauma-related mortality amongst illicit drug users (Davoli et al., 1997; Engstrom et al., 1991; Goedert et al., 1995; Maxwell et al., 2005; Perucci et al., 1991). Engstrom et al. (1991) reported a trauma-specific standardised mortality ratio (SMR) of 17.6, while Davoli et al. (1997) reported SMRs ranging between 4.0 and 15.5. Consistent with their levels of trauma exposure, death rates due to trauma among dependent drug users far exceed general population rates.

7.3 Demography of traumatic death

Amongst the general population, males are far more likely than females to be exposed to trauma (Hidalgo & Davidson, 2000; Kessler et al., 1995, Norris, 1992). There are, however, marked gender differences between the types of traumatic risk exposure experienced, with males more likely to experience physical assault, and females more likely to be sexually assaulted (Hidalgo & Davidson, 2000; Kessler et al., 1995; Norris, 1992). At a population level, males are also more likely to die from traumatic injury, including assault, falls, drownings, and MVAs (Australian Bureau of Statistics, 2003; Centers for Disease Control, 2003; Office of National Statistics, 2004).

This gender difference between types of trauma exposure is also seen amongst opioid users. Whilst male opioid users are more likely to have been physically assaulted, females are more likely to be the victim of sexual assault (Clark et al., 2001; Mills et al., 2005). It is unclear, however, whether there is any overall gender difference in trauma exposure between male and female drug users. PTSD has been shown to be higher amongst female opioid users compared to their male counterparts (Clark et al., 2001; Cottler et al., 1992; Mills et al., 2005). There are several possible explanations for this gender imbalance. Female opioid users may experience more traumatic incidents, there may be different levels of trauma associated with different traumatic events, or females may be more prone to experience PTSD. The answers to this issue are beyond the scope of this book. The only study of drug users to have compared exposure to trauma amongst opiate users by gender, however, found equally high proportions of both genders had experienced a traumatic event (Mills et al., 2005).

Few studies of illicit drug users have reported traumatic death rates by gender (Table 7.2). As has been found with overall mortality, the trauma-specific SMRs of female drug users are higher than those of males (Davoli et al., 1997; Engstrom et al., 1991). Female cohort members are thus more likely to die from traumatic injury than non-drug using female peers, than are males compared to non-drug using males. As with overall mortality, however, this does necessarily mean female drug users die from trauma at a rate greater than male drug users. In fact, what stands out from an inspection of Table 7.2 is the *similarity* in the proportions of traumatic fatalities amongst both genders (e.g. 5% versus 6%, Bartu et al., 2004; 8% versus 9%, Galli & Musicco, 1994; 12% versus 11%, Maxwell et al., 2005). These data are consistent with the only study to have reported rates of traumatic death by gender, which reported rates of 2.1 per thousand person-years amongst both male and female cohort members (Galli & Musicco, 1994). Higher female illicit drug user SMRs thus appears to reflect lower base rates of traumatic mortality amongst females in the general population, rather than a lower mortality rate compared to male drug users.

Why are rates of traumatic death amongst dependent female illicit drug users as high as those of male drug users, when rates of trauma and traumatic death in the general population rates are higher among males? The answer to this would appear to lie in the risks associated with illicit drug use per se. As noted above, the scope for conflict and violence in such circumstances is high. In addition, street sex work is common amongst dependent female drug users which, by its very nature, carries a high degree of physical risk. Driving motor vehicles whilst intoxicated with illicit drugs is also a widespread problem amongst both genders, and accident rates amongst drug users are substantially higher than those of the general population (Darke et al., 2003a). Violence and paranoia are also strongly associated with the use of psychostimulant drugs such as cocaine, regardless of gender. The lifestyle that revolves around dependent drug use thus carries a high degree of trauma risk that appears to be equivalent for persons of either gender.

7.4   Types of traumatic death

7.4.1   *Motor vehicle accidents*

Substance use appears to be a major contributor to MVA trauma. Internationally, studies report alcohol in excess of legal limits in 10–50%, and of other drugs between 5% and 30%, of accident involved drivers (cf. Kelly et al., 2004). The

Table 7.2. Trauma as a cause of death amongst illicit drug users by gender

Study	Country/period	Sample	Drug	Proportion of deaths due to trauma	
				Males (%)	Females (%)
Bartu et al. (2003)	Australia 1985–1998	Hospital/psychiatric admissions	Opioids, amphetamine	5	6
Benson & Holmberg (1984)	Sweden 1968–1978	Conscripts, rehabilitation & psychiatric patients, welfare recipients	Cannabis, solvents, LSD, stimulants	35	29
Cherubin et al. (1972)	USA 1964–1968	Notified addicts	Heroin	6	9
Davoli et al. (1997)	Italy 1980–1992	Treatment	IDU	16	8
Darke et al. (2005a)	Australia 1993–2002	Coronial	Cocaine	2	4
Dukes et al. (1992)	New Zealand 1971–1989	Treatment	Opioids	9	10
Galli & Musicco (1994)	Italy 1980–1991	Treatment	Methadone	8	9
Gill et al. (2002)	USA 1997–2000	Coronial	MDMA	33	0
Maxwell et al. (2005)	USA 1994–2002	Deaths in methadone	Opioids	12	11
Miotto et al. (1997)	USA	Treatment	Heroin	0	0
Oppenheimer et al. (1994)	UK 1969–1991	Treatment	Heroin	11	8
Perucci et al. (1991)	Italy 1980–1988	Treatment	Opioids	23	10
Tunving (1988)	Sweden 1970–1984	Treatment	Opioids, amphetamine	13	10
Webb et al. (2003)	UK 2000	Drug-related deaths	All	3	2
Zanis & Woody (1998)	USA 1993–1994	Methadone	Heroin	0	0
Zhu et al. (2000)	Japan 1994–1998	Coronial	Amphetamine	60	40

most commonly detected drugs, other than alcohol, among fatal MVA victims are cannabis, benzodiazepines, cocaine, amphetamines, and opioids (Athanaselis et al., 1999; Drummer et al., 2003; Gjerde et al., 1993; Jones & Holmgren, 2005; Kelly et al., 2004; Longo et al., 2000; Marzuk et al., 1990; Seymour & Oliver, 1999; Sjogren et al., 1997). Consistent with the polydrug use of illicit drug users, multiple drug detection is common, and 5–20% of killed or injured drivers have alcohol/drug combinations detected. Cannabis has played a relatively small role in this book in relation to overdose, disease, and suicide. It is apparent from these fatality figures, however, that cannabis plays a prominent role in MVA.

The mere presence of drugs does not prove evidence for a causal role in these accidents. Evidence from laboratory and simulator studies, however, confirms the role of drugs and alcohol. There is unequivocal evidence that alcohol produces significant impairment in driving performance (Hindmarch et al., 1991; Kelly et al., 2004; Robbe & Hanlon, 1999). Similarly, laboratory studies have generally found decreased psychomotor performance due to benzodiazepines (Busto et al., 2000; Mintzer & Griffiths, 1999; O'Neill et al., 2000). Importantly, there is evidence from laboratory, simulator, and driving studies that cannabis significantly impairs driving performance (Ashton, 1999; Drummer et al., 2003; European Monitoring Centre for Drugs and Drug Addiction, 1999a; Kelly et al., 2004; O'Kane et al., 2002; Robbe et al., 1999; Walsh et al., 2004). It is well known that opioid administration induces mental clouding and drowsiness (Walker et al., 2001). There is some evidence that low doses of psychostimulants may actually enhance performance in some psychomotor tasks, but only in fatigued subjects performing simple tasks, of which driving is clearly not one (Cami et al., 2000; Ellinwood & Nikaido, 1987; European Monitoring Centre for Drugs and Drug Addiction, 1999a).

Few studies have examined the prevalence of drug driving amongst illicit drug users (Aitken et al., 2000; Albery et al., 2000; Blomberg & Preusser, 1974; Darke et al., 2003a; Jones et al., 2005). Consistent with the toxicological data, these studies indicate that drug intoxicated driving, and drug intoxicated MVAs, are common. Albery et al. (2000) found 82% of illicit drug users had driven after consuming illicit drugs in the past year, most commonly heroin and/or cannabis, and a fifth had experienced a drug intoxicated accident in that period. Aitken et al. (2000) reported that two-thirds of injecting drug user (IDU) drivers had driven in the preceding week shortly after injecting drugs, and that a third had injected drugs shortly before their most recent MVA. Darke et al. (2003a) reported that 88% of IDU drivers had drug driven in the previous year (most commonly after using cannabis, heroin, amphetamines or cocaine),

Table 7.3. Death due to motor vehicle accident amongst illicit drug users

Study	Country/period	MVA (%)	Crude accident mortality rate (per 1000 person years)
Benson & Holmberg (1984)	Sweden 1968–1978	16	0.7
Bentley & Busuttil (1996)	UK 1989–1994	2	n/a
Darke et al. (2005a)	Australia 1993–2002	0	n/a
Dukes et al. (1992)	New Zealand 1980–1991	0	0
Galli & Musicco (1994)	Italy 1980–1991	4	1.0
Gill et al. (2002)	USA 1997–2000	9	n/a
Gronbladh et al. (1990)	Sweden 1967–1988	1	0.3
Logan et al. (1998)	USA 1993–1995	14	n/a
Maxwell et al. (2005)	USA 1994–2002	6	n/a
O'Doherty & Farrington (1997)	UK 1986–1991	5	n/a
Oppenheimer et al. (1994)	UK 1969–1991	0	0
Oyefesso et al. (1999b)	UK 1974–1993	1	0.1
Quaglio et al. (2001)	Italy 1985–1998	9	–
Raikos et al. (2002)	Greece 1998–2000	0	n/a
Zhu et al. (2000)	Japan 1994–1998	0	n/a

and a third had experienced a drug driving accident. As would be expected, given the effects of drugs on driving performance, the accident rate was 17 times that of the general population. Importantly, 15% had been injured while drug driving. Finally, Jones et al. (2005) reported that three quarters of cannabis users had driven after using cannabis in the preceding 12 months, and a quarter did so at least weekly.

Illicit drugs clearly have a strong association with psychomotor impairment, MVA injury, and death. Whilst not often reported separately from other trauma, cohort and coronial studies give some indication of the impact of MVAs on drug user mortality (Table 7.3). In most studies deaths due to road trauma represents a major component of overall trauma fatalities. Quaglio et al. (2001), for instance, reported road trauma as the third most common cause of death, with one in 10 deaths attributable to MVA. In very few studies was it possible to calculate crude mortality rates directly due to MVA: 1.0 per thousand person-years (Galli & Musicco, 1994), 0.7 per thousand person-years (Benson & Holmberg, 1984), 0.3 per thousand person-years (Gronbladh et al., 1990), and 0.05 per thousand person-years (Oyefesso et al., 1999b). By contrast, the mortality rate due to MVA in the general population is in the order of 0.1 per thousand

(Australian Bureau of Statistics, 2004; Centers for Disease Control, 2003; Office of National Statistics, 2004).

Males represent the majority of MVA deaths at a population level (Australian Bureau of Statistics, 2004; Centers for Disease Control, 2003; Office of National Statistics, 2004). Only two illicit drug user cohort studies have reported road trauma by gender (Benson & Holmberg, 1984; Quaglio et al., 2001). As with overall traumatic death, however, there was no difference between males and females in deaths due to MVA (16% versus 14%, Benson & Holmberg, 1984; 10% versus 8%, Quaglio et al., 2001). This is consistent with recent findings that drug driving is as common amongst female drug users as amongst males (Darke et al., 2003a).

7.4.2   *Other accidents*

The impairments in psychomotor performance, alertness, and judgement noted in relation to driving also have implications for accidents due to other causes. Impairment due to intoxication with illicit drugs may well increase the risk of fatal accidents due to falls from heights, drowning, etc. As with MVA and homicide fatalities, illicit drugs are commonly detected in non-MVA trauma victims (Copeland, 1984; Gill, 2001; Gill & Catanese, 2002; Lucas et al., 2002; Marzuk et al., 1995; Pachar & Cameron, 1992; Turk & Tsokos, 2004). By way of example, Turk & Tsokos (2004) reported one in 10 accidental fatal falls from heights as positive for morphine or cocaine, while a quarter of similar fatalities in Gill (2001) were positive for cocaine. Similarly high proportions have been found for accidental drowning (Copeland, 1984; Lucas et al., 2002; Pachar & Cameron, 1992), occupational fatalities (Greenberg et al., 1999), and accidental sharp object injuries (Gill & Catanese, 2002).

The proportion of deaths caused by non-MVA trauma amongst illicit drug users has not often been reported in cohort studies, or in retrospective studies of drug user deaths (Table 7.4). Where it has, the data has been consistent with the studies of accident victims and retrospective studies of illicit drug user deaths in suggesting that non-MVA trauma plays a significant role in illicit drug-related mortality (Table 7.4). The deaths in these studies include drowning, death due to falls, death from burns, etc. The crude non-MVA mortality rate in cohort studies ranges from 0 to 1.6 per thousand person-years. In half of these studies the rate exceeded 0.5 per thousand person-years. In comparison, in the USA the rate of death due to accidents is 0.4 per thousand, but this includes MVAs (Centers for Disease Control, 2003). Consistent with the relationship between drug use and accidents reported above, the rates of death due to non-MVA trauma appears to far exceed that of the general population.

Table 7.4. Death due to accidents other than motor vehicle accident amongst illicit drug users

Study	Country/period	Accidents (%)	Crude accident mortality rate (per 1000 person years)
Bartu et al. (2004)	Australia 1985–1998	4	0.1
Benson & Holmberg (1984)	Sweden 1968–1978	14	0.6
Bentley & Busutill (1996)	UK 1989–1994	3	n/a
Bucknall & Robertson (1986)	UK 1981–1985	0	0.0
Darke et al. (2005a)	Australia 1993–2002	3	n/a
Dukes et al. (1992)	New Zealand 1971–1989	4	0.3
Gill et al. (2002)	USA 1997–2000	18	n/a
Langendam et al. (2001)	Holland 1985–1996	1	0.3
Logan et al. (1998)	USA 1993–1995	29	n/a
Maxwell et al. (2005)	USA 1994–2002	1	n/a
O'Doherty & Farrington (1997)	UK 1986–1991	5	n/a
Oppenheimer et al. (1994)	UK 1969–1991	7	1.1
Oyefesso et al. (1999b)	UK 1974–1993	3	0.1
Raikos et al. (2002)	Greece 1998–2000	86	n/a
Tunving (1988)	Sweden 1970–1984	5	0.6
Vaillant (1973)	USA 1952–1970	2	0.2
Vlahov et al. (2004)	USA 1988–2000	3	1.0
Wille (1981)	UK 1969–1979	10	1.5
Zador & Sunjic (2000)	Australia 1990–1995	8	n/a
Zaccarelli et al. (1994)	Italy 1985–1991	7	1.6
Zhu et al. (2000)	Japan 1994–1998	33	n/a

7.4.3 Homicide

As noted above, the use of illicit drugs such as opiates and psychostimulants is strongly associated with crime and sex work, committed in order to support the drug habit. These activities carry a high risk of violence, particularly considering the large amounts of money involved, and the desperation of dependent users to obtain drugs. Consistent with this profile, as discussed above, reported rates of serious assault amongst dependent drug users are extremely high, and far exceed those amongst non-drug users (Clark et al., 2001; Mills et al., 2005).

Given this overall picture, death due to homicide or violence might be expected to play a significant role in illicit drug user deaths. Such, indeed, appears to be the case (Gill & Catanese, 2002; Gill et al., 2002, 2003; Harruff et al., 1988;

Table 7.5. Death due to homicide amongst illicit drug users

Study	Country/period	Homicide (%)	Crude homicide mortality rate (per 1000 person years)
Bartu et al. (2003)	Australia 1985–1998	2	0.04
Benson & Holmberg (1984)	Sweden 1968–1978	0	0.0
Bewley et al. (1968)	UK 1947–1966	9	2.4
Bucknall & Robertson (1986)	UK 1981–1985	14	1.4
Cooncool et al. (1979)	USA 1969–1976	38	2.1
Darke et al. (2005a)	Australia 1993–2002	0	n/a
Engstrom et al. (1991)	Sweden 1973–1984	4	0.9
Eskild et al. (1993)	Norway 1985–1991	4	0.9
Fugelstad et al. (1997)	Sweden 1981–1992	3	0.5
Galli & Musicco (1994)	Italy 1980–1991	5	1.3
Gill et al. (2002)	USA 1997–2000	5	n/a
Gossop et al. (2002b)	UK 1995–1999	14	1.1
Gronbladh et al. (1990)	Sweden 1967–1988	1	0.3
Karch et al. (1999)	USA 1985–1997	10	n/a
Logan et al. (1998)	USA 1993–1995	27	n/a
Maxwell et al. (2005)	USA 1994–2002	4	n/a
Oppenheimer et al. (1994)	UK 1969–1991	1	0.2
Orti et al. (1996)	Spain	12	3.6
Oyefesso et al. (1999b)	UK 1974–1993	0	0.0
Raikos et al. (2002)	Greece 1998–2000	0	n/a
Shaw (1999)	Taiwan 1991–1996	14	n/a
Tunving (1988)	Sweden 1970–1984	3	0.4
Wille (1981)	UK 1969–1979	0	0.0
Zador & Sunjic (2000)	Australia 1990–1995	5	n/a
Zaccarelli et al. (1994)	Italy 1985–1991	2	0.5
Zhu et al. (2000)	Japan 1994–1998	27	n/a

Karch et al., 1999; Rogers, 1993; Spunt et al., 1994, 1995; Tardiff et al., 2005; Zhu et al., 2000). As many as a third of homicide offenders are positive for illicit drugs and/or alcohol at the time of their offence (Spunt et al., 1994, 1995). Of central interest here, however, is the fact that large proportions of homicide victims are positive for illicit drugs (Gill & Catanese, 2002; Gill et al., 2003; Harruff et al., 1988; Rogers, 1993; Tardiff et al., 2005). Over a 9-year period, 28% of in New York homicide victims were positive for cocaine, 19% for cannabis, and 11% for opiates (Tardiff et al., 2005). Similar or even higher figures have been reported in other studies (Gill & Catanese, 2002; Gill et al., 2003; Harruff et al., 1988; Marzuk et al., 1995; Rogers, 1993). Moreover, a recent study reported that the overall homicide rate in New York covaried with the rate of homicide cases that were positive for cocaine (Tardiff et al., 2005).

Only a minority of cohort and coronial studies of illicit drug users deaths have specifically reported homicide independent of other types of traumatic death (Table 7.5). As can be seen from Table 7.5, and consistent with the above studies, those studies report homicide amongst substantial proportions of fatalities, ranging as high as 38% (Cooncool et al., 1979). The mortality rates of illicit drug using cohorts appear to far exceed population rates. For instance, the mortality rates due to homicide in the USA are 0.06 per thousand, 0.01 per thousand in the UK/Europe, and 0.02 per thousand in Australia (Australian Bureau of Statistics, 2004; Centers for Disease Control, 2003; Office of National Statistics, 2004). By contrast, in almost all cases, the incidence rates in the cohort studies far exceed these rates (Table 7.5).

7.5   Summary of trauma and illicit drug use

PTSD and life-threatening events are common amongst opioid and cocaine users, and occur at levels considerably higher than amongst non-drug users. Serious physical assault in particular, appears extremely common. Consistent with their higher rates of trauma exposure, mortality rates amongst illicit drug users due to trauma exceed those of the general population. The major causes of traumatic death amongst illicit drug users are MVA, non-MVA trauma, and homicide. Illicit drugs are commonly detected amongst fatalities due to each of these forms of trauma, and all occur amongst illicit drug users at rates exceeding those of the general population. Despite the salience of the issue demonstrated in this chapter, trauma is by far the least studied or recognised cause of death amongst illicit drug users. In Chapters 8 and 9 we present recommendations for intervention and research to redress this imbalance.

Key points: Summary of trauma and illicit drug use

- Rates of PTSD are significantly higher amongst illicit drug users than non-drug users.
- Life-threatening events, and serious physical assault in particular, are common amongst users of illicit drugs, particularly opioids and cocaine.
- Most cohort studies report mortality rates exceeding 2.0 per thousand person-years, compared to 0.04 per thousand amongst the general population.
- Major causes of traumatic death amongst illicit drug users are MVA, other accidents, and homicide.
- Illicit drugs have deleterious effects upon psychomotor performance and judgment.
- Substance use is a major contributor to MVA trauma. The most commonly detected illicit drug is cannabis.
- Illicit drugs are frequently detected amongst homicide victims, and homicide rates amongst illicit drug users far exceed those of the general population.
- Illicit drugs are frequently detected amongst non-MVA trauma victims, and non-MVA trauma rates amongst illicit drug users far exceed those of the general population.

8

Reducing drug-related mortality

8.1 Introduction

The preceding chapters have presented detailed analyses of the major causes of illicit drug-related mortality, as well as the demographic characteristics of drug-related fatalities, possible mechanisms, and risk factors for such deaths. In this chapter we examine various means of reducing such deaths. Some interventions are well established, such as the various treatment modalities for opioid dependence. Others have been proposed, but have yet to be implemented and/or evaluated. The area of drug-related traumatic injury has not been addressed at all by intervention, so any discussion is necessarily speculative.

8.2 Drug treatment

As noted in Chapter 3, drug-dependence treatment has a substantial role in reducing mortality and morbidity associated with illicit drug use. This is especially true in the context of opioid dependence, the drug class associated with the greatest risk of death (cf. Chapter 3). The strongest, and largest body, of research in this regard comes from studies of methadone-maintenance treatment (and other opioid replacement therapies), and its effect on drug-injecting behaviour and mortality rates. This is not, of course, to suggest that retention in other forms of long-term treatment, such as drug-free residential rehabilitation, do not reduce risk of death. Indeed, long-term retention in both maintenance and residential rehabilitation have been demonstrated to reduce the risk of non-fatal heroin overdose (Darke et al., 2005f; Stewart et al., 2002), and thus the risk of one of the major killers of opioid users. This section, however, will focus on opioid maintenance therapies, as these have been the most extensively researched. To date, there are no effective pharmacotherapies for the treatment of cocaine, amphetamine, or methylenedioxymethamphetamine (MDMA) dependence.

Opioid replacement therapy, and methadone maintenance in particular, has been demonstrated to reduce mortality (Brugal et al., 2005; Caplehorn et al., 1994; Gronbladh et al., 1990; Ward et al., 1992, 1998, 1999). It is less clear that treatment for other (non-opioid) illicit drug use decreases death rates, partly because of a lack of systematic evidence. Methadone has been consistently shown to reduce the rate of opioid injecting (Mattick et al., 2003a). This effect has two direct benefits. First, it reduces exposure to illicit opioids, and hence the possibility of overdose from ingestion of heroin. Second, it reduces exposure to blood-borne viral infections (BBVI), and hence to death associated with disease. Although methadone itself can be toxic if prescribed at too high a dose, or used by those for whom it was not intended, or where tolerance is limited (Buster et al., 2002; Drummer et al., 1990, 1992), it is protective of health and reduces mortality from many causes amongst opioid dependent persons. The evidence of this effect comes mainly from observational studies, as the randomised clinical trials of treatment have typically been of too short a duration, and samples sizes too small to allow for detection of effects on mortality (Amato et al., 2005; Mattick et al. 2003a, b).

8.2.1   Early evidence of methadone treatment preventing death

Although there was preliminary evidence from researchers in the US that methadone reduced mortality (Gearing & Schweitzer, 1974), it was researchers in Sweden (Gronbladh et al., 1990) who provided the first convincing evidence of a reduction in mortality rates. They took advantage of a natural experiment. After the establishment of a methadone programme in Sweden between 1967 and 1988 (Grönbladh & Gunne, 1989), entry of new patients to methadone was not possible for the years 1979–1984. The yearly death rates over the 5–8-year period of observation from any cause in a cohort of heroin-dependent individuals showed that for those in methadone treatment (MT), 1.40% died per annum. For "successful" graduates of methadone, 1.7% died, whereas 6.9% of those patients who were involuntarily discharged from treatment died, and 7.2% of patients who were provided "intermittent detoxification and participated in drug-free treatment" died annually. These authors reported that deaths while in MT were still 8.4 times greater than expected compared with general population rates, but those involuntarily discharged from methadone had a death rate 55.3 times greater than expected, and those receiving detoxification or drug-free services had a death rate 63.1 times greater than expected. Interestingly, of those in MT who died, many deaths were due to pre-existing physical illness (and therefore not attributable to methadone), and none were caused by methadone overdose. Of the deaths that occurred outside methadone, 71% were attributed to heroin overdose (partly or totally). This last result is, of course, consistent with methadone being protective against heroin overdose due to cross-tolerance to other opioid drugs (so that a person tolerant to a given dose of heroin will show tolerance to an equipotent dose of methadone or another opioid) (Jaffe & Martin, 1985).

Put simply, this study demonstrated that methadone reduced rates of over-dose and some other health complications. Gronbladh et al. (1990) described the causes of death of those who died in MT. These simple and brief descriptions bring into sharp focus the data presented elsewhere herein about some of the causes of death among injecting drug users and are salutary about the range of health problems faced by these people, even when in effective MT:

"Many of these [methadone] patients had potentially fatal diseases when they entered the MT program. Three were alcoholics, 2 with impaired liver function, in 1 case leading to ruptured esophageal varicosities. Another case of cirrhosis posthepatitis was not an alcoholic, but died of liver coma. One subject had an esophageal stricture caused by accidentally swallowing lye in childhood. He feared the monthly painful probing and distension treatments, which made him an iatrogenic morphine addict. In the end he took an overdose of barbiturates. Three patients had acquired severe heart damage through repeated bacterial infections of the endo- and myocardium. One patient, a former amphetamine addict, after 11 years of successful rehabilitation, met an old amphetamine-addicted friend. They decided to take a dose of amphetamine together and the patient died from a ruptured arterial brain aneurysm.

In addition to severe acquired diseases, some of these [deceased methadone] subjects had mental handicaps, rendering their rehabilitation difficult. Three had difficulties reading and writing ... [and] one woman had ... displayed signs of periodic depression, which may have contributed to her eventual suicide. One death from overdose was judged by police to be murder. This patient had received threatening telephone calls from a drug dealer, who claimed that the patient owed him money. He was found dead, beaten up in the streets, with a syringe beside him" (p. 226).

Gronbladh et al. (1990) also described barriers to rehabilitation preceding death in their methadone patients. This description is instructive as it indicates how negative attitudes of health professional and society to this treatment can potentially compromise the effectiveness of methadone, a problem separately argued by Ball with regard to methadone programs broadly (Ball & Ross, 1991):

"... In one instance the staff of a vocational training centre demanded our patient be taken off methadone or be excluded from the training program. After that we did not manage to find him a job and soon afterwards he committed suicide. A female patient one day found, when she came home from work, that her brother (also a drug addict) had hung himself in the kitchen. After that she had difficulties sleeping and asked for psychotherapy, "just someone to talk to". We tried to arrange such a contact … but it turned out to be impossible. Our psychiatric colleagues refused to talk to her unless she would first agree to have her methadone discontinued (which she did not dare). She lost her job and was sent to a vocational training centre where the staff had her expelled due to MT. She then had problems with her fiancé, who maltreated her, and in the end this woman committed suicide. Another patient, a man with reading difficulties, was unable to find a job for a couple of years. Finally he was hired as a caretaker by one of the societies for drug addicts. Since they were opposed to MT he kept his treatment a secret, but was eventually found out and fired. He returned to unemployment, took up abuse of sedatives and finally died from myocarditis.

Although the mortality within MT was low compared with our controls, there were thus several complex reasons for some continuing mortality once within the programme" (p. 226).

Taken together, the results of Gronbladh et al. (1990) showed that MT protected patients against premature death due to heroin overdose (cf. Chapter 4), and that its effectiveness was partly mediated by the adequacy of treatment and ancillary services. In Italy, the same effect was independently observed (Davoli et al., 1993), and the authors concluded that a "high risk of overdose death occurred among subjects who left treatment compared with those still in treatment" (p. 273).

Buprenorphine has yet to be fully examined in this regard, but it should have similar benefits to methadone, and it is notable that the recent Kakko et al. (2003) study showed an excess of deaths in placebo-maintained patients compared with buprenorphine-treated patients. Moreover, the results from the major randomised trials of buprenorphine show a strong effect similar to that of methadone, albeit with slightly less retention (Ling et al., 1996; Mattick et al., 2003a, b; Strain et al., 1994a, b).

8.2.2   Studies supporting the effect of methadone on reducing mortality

Subsequent to the early work in Sweden, others have shown that retention in methadone is associated with reduced mortality. Caplehorn et al. (1994) in Australia were able to demonstrate that patients were 3 times as likely to die outside methadone as in it. Moreover, they showed that higher doses of methadone were associated with better outcome. Subsequently, Caplehorn et al. (1996) drew on a number of studies to provide evidence that enrolment in MT reduced mortality risk by nearly 75%.

In the USA, a study of patients who entered MT showed that death rates, especially opioid overdose deaths, were more frequent among those who were "unfavourably discharged" or who dropped out of MT (Zanis & Woody, 1998). The authors opined that "at-risk" patients should be maintained in treatment even if their treatment response was suboptimal. The same effects were noted among Australian prisoners (Dolan et al., 2005).

The protective effect of methadone has also been observed by other investigators in different settings: being in MT has been shown to reduce the rate of opioid overdose. Esteban et al. (2003) studied patients who received MT in Spain in the 1990s, and found that being in treatment significantly predicted improved survival. Similarly, Brugal and colleagues from Spain demonstrated that an observed decline in mortality was related to the effects of MT on overdose rates (Brugal et al., 2005). This effect seems to be dose related with higher doses being more protective in preventing overdose death than lower doses (van Ameijden et al., 1999b), a finding consistent with that reported by others (Caplehorn et al., 1994). Of course, this finding is consistent with the fact that higher methadone doses reduce heroin use better than lower doses (Ward et al., 1992, 1998, 1999), and that higher methadone doses will provide a greater level of tolerance and cross-tolerance to other opioids. Indeed, a high dose of methadone produces more tolerance, and therefore it is more difficult to overdose on opioids. In fact, the high blockade doses (above 100 mg) of methadone are so effective that there is reportedly very little effect from ingesting further opioids, and little chance of a toxic result (Dole et al., 1966; Jaffe, 1985; Kreek, 1983, 1987).

8.2.3 Role of pharmacotherapies in preventing HIV seroconversion and death

In the late 1980s the first published reports showing the effectiveness of methadone maintenance treatment in preventing human immunodeficiency virus (HIV) infection appeared. In New York, HIV infection had spread rapidly among injecting drug users between the late 1970s and early 1980s (Des Jarlais et al., 1989). In one of the initial studies attesting to the effect of methadone on reducing HIV seroconversion, Abdul-Quader et al. (1987) reported an association between lower rates of HIV antibody and length of time enrolled in MT. Soon thereafter, Schoenbaum et al. (1989) showed the same result. Around that time, Novick et al. (1990) also reported that there was no evidence of exposure to HIV amongst a group of stable patients who had remained in long-term treatment, and two further studies from the USA then showed that there was greater likelihood of HIV infection in those in detoxification (Marmor et al., 1987) or not yet in MT (Chaisson et al., 1989), compared with those receiving MT.

These early studies were, however, observational, and other factors such as motivation to reduce use could have explained the apparent benefit attributed to methadone. They were not as convincing as the randomised studies that came later. Again, the Swedes took advantage of the relative inaccessibility of MT in their country to examine the effects of entering, or not entering, MT in what appears to have approximated a quasi-randomised study (Blix & Gronbladh, 1991; Blix & Grönbladh, 1988). The Blix and Gronbladh research relied on the fact that nearly all of the patients who entered treatment in Sweden after 1983 had previously applied for, and been refused, entry to such treatment. Refusal of entry was virtually random, as it relied on whether there was a place available, and not patient characteristics. What Blix and Gronbladh reported was that only 3% of patients who entered MT prior to 1983 were HIV-positive, whereas 16% of those entering treatment between 1984 and 1986 were positive, and 57% of those who entered treatment after 1986 were HIV-positive. Additionally, seroprevalence for those outside MT continued at 40% or more up until 1990, but no patient who tested negative for HIV at entry to MT seroconverted thereafter. This study provided strong evidence that methadone protects against HIV infection and that this is not simply a phenomenon associated with the types of patients who are willing to enter MT.

Subsequent to this evidence being published, a series of cohort studies supported the Swedish observations. In the USA, Metzger et al. (1993) reported on regular opioid injectors sampled in- and out-of-treatment, who were followed over a 3-year period. The prevalence of HIV-positive results increased from 21% to 39% for the out-of-treatment group. In contrast, those in-treatment at the start of the study showed a smaller increase, from 13% to 18%. Of most interest, in the current context, was the finding that the 5% increase in sero-conversion was accounted for by those who left treatment.

The literature on the role of substitution therapies in the prevention of HIV infection has grown enormously over the past decade. There is now strong evidence that opioid substitution reduces injection-related risk behaviour among injecting opioid users, both in the community and in prisons (Dolan et al., 2003; Gowing et al., 2004). This reduction in risk behaviour is reflected in the findings of a number of independent researchers on different continents that enrolment in opioid-maintenance treatment protects against HIV infection (Abdul-Quader et al., 1987; Blix & Gronbladh, 1991; Blix & Grönbladh, 1988; Brown et al., 1989; Chaisson et al., 1989; Marmor et al., 1987; Metzger et al.,

1993; Schoenbaum et al., 1989). Given the evidence of similar effects of methadone and buprenorphine (cf. 8.2.4), the protective effect should also be exerted by buprenorphine maintenance treatment (Ward et al., 1998), and recent evidence shows reduced injecting behaviours among HIV-positive opioid-dependent patients in buprenorphine maintenance (Carrieri et al., 2003).

8.2.4 Buprenorphine maintenance

As noted earlier, buprenorphine is an effective medication for maintenance therapy. There is now evidence that buprenorphine used with HIV-positive patients can ease opioid withdrawal symptoms (Montoya et al., 1995; Umbricht et al., 2003), and also evidence which suggests that buprenorphine can protect against HIV seroconversion (Duburcq et al., 2000). It should be noted that, unlike buprenorphine, methadone can present a clinical problem in the management of some HIV-positive opioid users, as it apparently interacts with HIV-related medications (Gourevitch & Friedland, 2000). This is a difficulty for methadone maintenance therapy in patients being treated for HIV/AIDS, as adverse drug interactions between methadone and antiretroviral agents make management more difficult. Some of the pharmacokinetic and pharmacodynamic interactions of buprenorphine with a range of antiretroviral agents, however, have been studied. There is evidence that while methadone interacts adversely with zidovudine (McCance-Katz et al., 1998), buprenorphine does not show an increase in zidovudine concentrations, and thus produces fewer adverse effects (McCance-Katz et al., 2002).

This potential for adverse drug interactions from medications (or illicit drugs) ingested while in methadone maintenance treatment is addressed elsewhere (Ward et al., 1998). Many other drugs can adversely complicate management with methadone by affecting liver metabolism. More recent findings, for example, show that opioid-dependent drug users suffering from HIV frequently suffer a severe opioid withdrawal syndrome when managed with highly active antiretroviral therapy (HAART) regimens which involve efavirenz (McCance-Katz et al., 2002). This withdrawal apparently occurs because the drug efavirenz induces cytochrome P450 3A4, the enzyme chiefly responsible for the metabolism of methadone. It is possible that buprenorphine will simplify the treatment of opioid-dependent patients who are medicated with efavirenz. Similarly, methadone has been associated with opiate abstinence symptoms when administered in combination with lopinavir/ritonavir (McCance-Katz et al., 2002). Buprenophine may prove superior to methadone in the management of HIV-positive patients.

8.2.5   Naltrexone treatment

Naltrexone is opioid antagonist which, if taken in regular maintenance doses, suppresses the effects of opioids. There is little evidence that naltrexone is an effective treatment for the management of opioid dependence. There is evidence, however, of some value for a minority of patients who are willing to enter and remain in the treatment (Kirchmayer et al., 2002; Minozzi et al., 2001, 2006). The evidence from randomised trials to date, however, is flawed and weak. The general conclusion drawn is that oral naltrexone has been, and will remain, a minority option for the management of opioid dependence. As such, it is unlikely to play a major role in the prevention of opioid-related death, from a broad public health perspective. Additionally, there is some evidence of increased rates of overdose among patients soon after leaving this treatment (arguably due to the loss of opioid tolerance) (Digiusto et al., 2004). It should be noted that the new implantable depot formulations of naltrexone may well improve compliance and reduce overdose risk. This, however, remains to be demonstrated in randomised controlled trials.

8.2.6   Treatment of other drug use problems

The value of treatment in reducing seroconversion to HIV for opioid injectors can easily be realised in the context of other drug types, if such users are drawn into treatment that is effective, and reduces risky injecting. The literature to date, however, is not as strong for the treatment of psychostimulant, or other non-opioid, drug problems. To the extent that treatment reduces injecting drug use, there should be a corresponding effect in terms of the impact on both injecting and exposure to risk behaviours associated with HIV seroconversion.

8.3   Treatment of blood-borne viral infections

As noted in Chapter 5, rates of hepatitis C (HCV) among injecting drug users (IDU) are high worldwide, and in many countries HIV prevalence rates are considerably elevated compared to the general population. These illnesses have been shown to account for significant morbidity and mortality among IDU. Fortunately, effective treatment options do exist for both HCV and HIV.

In the case of HCV, recent years have seen significant developments in the treatment of the illness. These include interferon monotherapy, combination interferon, and ribavirin and pegylated or interferon which provides sustained delivery of the agent (Manns et al., 2001; McHutchinson et al., 1998; Poynard, 2004). Such treatments have been found to eradicate HCV in a significant proportion of patients, and reduce the onset of liver cirrhosis (Poynard, 2004).

In the case of HIV, HAART has been shown to lead to reductions in HIV viral load, in deaths related to HIV/AIDS, and to improve quality of life among varied populations of HIV-positive persons (Chesney et al., 2000; Ellis et al., 2003; Murphy et al., 2002; Vlahov et al., 2005). The reduction in viral HIV load associated with HAART carries implications for risk of transmission between IDU through injecting as well as through sexual transmission (Castilla et al., 2005). One study suggested that following the introduction of HAART, a reduction of approximately 80% in heterosexual transmission of HIV was observed, irrespective of changes in other factors that are known to affect transmission risk (Castilla et al., 2005).

Co-infection of HIV and HCV is common (cf. Chapter 5). Recent reviews of the evidence have been consistent in their recommendations that persons with co-infection should receive treatment for both diseases (Poynard, 2004; Tien, 2005). However, the treatment of HCV in HIV/HCV co-infected patients can be complicated by the hepatotoxic effects of HIV medication, as well as by HIV infection itself (Tien, 2005). Immune levels need to be examined among HIV-positive persons before commencing HCV treatment.

Unfortunately, illicit drug users are under-represented among eligible persons receiving HIV and HCV treatment. One explanation for this may be the assumption that drug users are less capable than others of adhering to complicated medication regimens. Adherence to HAART promotes viral suppression and can significantly extend and improve the lives of persons with HIV (Casado et al., 1999; Chesney et al., 2000; Ellis et al., 2003). The difficulties of adhering consistently to HAART are significant because of the complexity of the regimens, the severity of medication side effects, and the need for 95% adherence to avoid development of drug resistance (Chesney et al., 2000). Poor adherence to HAART is associated with the development of resistance to antiretroviral drugs as well as to less-effective inhibition of viral replication (Chesney et al., 2000; Ellis et al., 2003).

There is evidence to suggest that problematic drug users do, in fact, have lower adherence levels (Ellis et al., 2003; Kerr et al., 2004; Lucas et al., 2001, 2002). One study in the US found that amongst HIV-positive men receiving treatment for methamphetamine dependence, methamphetamine was associated with "unplanned non-adherence" to HIV medication (Reback et al., 2003). This was distinct from "planned non-adherence" to treatment, whereby HIV-positive persons took a break from the schedules of HIV medication. Unplanned adherence was thought by participants to be the result of the impact of methamphetamine upon sleep and food intake (Reback et al., 2003). Work needs to be carried out to investigate the reasons for non-adherence, and to increase the coverage, and effectiveness, of treatments for BBVI among IDU.

8.4   Harm reduction

In this section we examine non-drug treatment interventions specifically aimed at reducing mortality from the major causes of illicit drug-related death. The extensive provision of drug-treatment programmes will in all probability provide the most effective, and politically feasible, means of reducing illicit drug-related mortality. A number of more specific interventions, however, have arisen from the literature and from clinical practice. These are broadly placed here under the rubric "harm reduction". It is important to note that these are not antithetical to the provision of drug treatment, and may well provide useful adjuncts for reducing drug-related mortality and morbidity.

8.4.1   Overdose

Education: The earlier chapter on overdose emphasised the strong role that is played by polydrug use in overdose fatalities. In particular, the concomitant use of heroin with other central nervous system (CNS) depressant drugs substantially increases the risk of death from overdose. Given this association, education of heroin users on the risks of polydrug use may help reduce the frequency of heroin overdose. Such information might be presented through treatment programmes, needle exchange programmes, and outreach services. Medical practitioners also clearly need to be aware of the role of prescribed medications such as benzodiazepines and tricyclic antidepressants in contributing to heroin overdose. Campaigns to improve awareness among heroin users have been conducted, but rarely evaluated. It has, however, been demonstrated that awareness of risk factors can be raised by means of such campaigns (McGregor et al., 2001). Changing the actual behaviours involved may be more difficult (McGregor et al., 2001). The increased risk associated with concomitant use of cocaine and heroin need to be emphasised to primary users of both of these drugs.

Polydrug use is also important for cocaine and amphetamine users. The role of alcohol, for instance, in increasing the toxicity of these drugs should be emphasised. Information on the cardiotoxic nature of these drugs is of paramount importance. It is unlikely that the effects of these drugs in causing heart disease are widely known by users. Given the demographics of these deaths and of coronary disease, older male users of these drugs would appear to be the major target group. The primary information directed at ecstasy users should concern the risks of hyperthermia and over-hydration. The risks of cardiovascular events and liver damage also need to be emphasised.

Education on the increased risk of overdosing when resuming heroin use after a period of abstinence is essential, especially for older users. The demographic and toxicological evidence discussed earlier on increased risk for older users (cf. Chapter 4) emphasises the importance of this group as an intervention target. This is also particularly relevant for heroin users about to be released from prison, a high-risk period for overdose (Chapter 4). Information on overdose risk could form a component of pre-release counselling about risks involved in resuming heroin use.

Overall, research into the provision of information on risk reduction to illicit drug users would appear to be a clinical and research priority. Such campaigns would not attempt to legitimise illicit drug use but, rather, attempt to reduce mortality amongst those at greatest risk of death. As noted above, there is limited research in a single jurisdiction to indicate that awareness of risk factors can be raised by means of such a campaign (McGregor et al., 2001). Given the salience of overdose, extensive international research into such interventions is well warranted.

Bystander responses to overdose are poor (Darke et al., 1996b, 2000; Davidson et al., 2003; Kaye & Darke, 2004; Manning et al., 1983; McGregor et al., 2001; Strang et al., 2000; Tracy et al., 2005). Drug user education should thus not only concentrate on reducing risk factors for overdose, but also on improving responses to overdose by other drug users who are present. This applies to users of any illicit drug, and may well prevent many avoidable deaths. For example, heroin users could be taught simple cardiopulmonary resuscitation skills so that they can keep comatose opioid users alive until help arrives (Dettmer et al., 2001; Galea et al., 2006; McGregor et al., 2001; Seal et al., 2005). Users of any drug also need to be encouraged to call an ambulance immediately after an overdose occurs. The understandable fears of police involvement need to be addressed. Encouragingly, amongst heroin users it has been demonstrated that such interventions can improve responses of witnesses to overdose, including performing cardiopulmonary resuscitation and calling ambulances (Dettmer et al., 2001; Galea et al., 2006; McGregor et al., 2001; Seal et al., 2005). In the McGregor et al. (2001) study, this occurred within a broader context in which ambulance officials and police agreed upon emergency protocols where police would not routinely attend overdose events, unless death or violence occurred. As with the provision of information on risk factors, trials on improving responses to overdose appear to be a research priority, given what is known about current responses.

Naloxone provision: A possible adjunct to education on improved responses to opioid overdoses in particular is the provision of naloxone hydrochloride directly to heroin users (Darke & Hall, 1997, 2003; Lenton & Hargreaves, 2000a, b; Strang et al., 1996, 2000). Naloxone hydrochloride is a narcotic antagonist that reverses the effects of acute narcosis, including respiratory depression, sedation, and hypotension. It can be administered by intravenous, intramuscular, subcutaneous, or intranasal routes (Darke & Hall, 1997; Leimer et al., 1994). If made widely available to heroin users, it could be distributed through existing outlets such as needle and syringe exchanges, pharmacies, general practitioners (GPs), or treatment agencies. The ampoules of naloxone would be stored in heroin users' homes for use in the event of an overdose, but would need to be refrigerated. The major potential advantage is the increased chance of a comatose opioid user being quickly resuscitated by others who are present. Logistical factors in favour of such an intervention include the fact that most heroin overdoses occur in home environments, heroin users are frequent witnesses to overdoses, and others are frequently present at overdoses (Darke et al., 1996b, 2000; Davidson et al., 2003; Kaye & Darke, 2004; Man et al., 2002; McGregor et al., 1998; Strang et al., 2000). Furthermore, naloxone has no pharmacological activity in the absence of opioids, and lacks abuse potential.

Any evaluation of this option would need to assess the seriousness of a number of potential problems. First, in almost all jurisdictions, there are medico-legal complications for medical practitioners prescribing a drug most likely to be administered to, and by, persons other than the one for whom it was prescribed (Darke & Hall, 2003; Lenton & Hargreaves, 2000b). There are also significant economic costs in distributing naloxone sufficiently widely to have a significant impact on overdose morbidity and mortality. On a more immediate clinical level, the half-life of naloxone is shorter than that of opioids, which means that the ability of naloxone to reverse the effects of opioids is of limited duration. Thus, a person whose narcosis has been reversed by naloxone can relapse into coma if the effects of the opioid persist beyond the half-life of naloxone. This risk can be overcome by the administration of further doses of naloxone.

While naloxone has been made available as an over the counter drug in Italy since 1995, and also provided more directly to heroin users, no formal evaluation has been conducted (Lenton & Hargreaves, 2000b; Simini, 1998). Small-scale pilot distribution schemes have been conducted in Germany, Jersey and the US, in conjunction with broader resuscitation training (Dettmer et al., 2001; Galea et al., 2006; Seal et al., 2005). While small in scale, these studies have indicated that heroin users will use naloxone appropriately, that they are able to reverse overdoses in emergency situations and that adverse effects do not appear to be a problem. Given the promising preliminary data, full trials into the efficacy of naloxone provision, and any associated problems, are well worth while. Again, it needs to be borne in mind that naloxone provision would not be a legitimization of opioid use, but an attempt to save lives amongst those at risk.

It is important to emphasise that there are no analogous antagonist drugs that could form the basis of peer interventions for toxicity due to cocaine, amphetamine, or MDMA.

Routes of administration: As discussed previously (Chapter 4), injecting is a risk factor for opioid overdose, and appears also to be so for cocaine and amphetamine. In relation to heroin, it has been suggested that interventions be designed to encourage users to switch to non-injecting routes of administration, thus reducing the risk of overdose (Hunt et al., 1999). One concern with such a policy is that it may increase the aggregate number of heroin users due to increased popularity of initiating use via a less "frightening" route of administration, before later moving to injection. It may, in the longer term, also increase the number of heroin injectors if substantial proportions of smokers make the transition to injecting, which is by far the more common transition (Darke et al., 2005b; Neaigus et al., 2001; Perez-Jimenez & Robert, 1997; Strang et al., 1999). Of more immediate issue is the question of practicality. Studies of transitions between routes of administration indicate that existing injectors are resistant to abandoning injecting. It would appear unlikely that large numbers of injectors would be willing, or indeed able, to change to alternative routes.

It should also be borne in mind that the long-term cardiotoxic effects of cocaine and amphetamines occurs irrespective of route of administration. Such effects relate to the drug itself, whilst heroin overdose is strongly related to the proximal route.

Medically supervised injecting centres: A more far more politically contentious intervention is the provision of medically supervised injecting centres. These are officially designated sites at which IDU can inject drugs without fear of arrest, and in the knowledge that medical assistance is available. Such an intervention is clearly not directed towards any one drug. Such facilities exist in Switzerland (since 1986), Germany (1994), and the Netherlands (1996), and a trial continues in Australia (Kimber et al., 2003). Evaluations of safe injecting

rooms have reported their acceptability to IDU, although their effect on overdose fatalities is still in debate (Dolan et al., 2000; Kimber et al., 2003). It must
be borne in mind that, as discussed above, the majority of overdoses occur in
the home environment. Such facilities would appear of greatest utility in reducing overdose fatalities in locations where there is a substantial degree of street-
based injecting.

8.4.2 Disease

The primary diseases related to illicit injecting drug use are due to BBVI,
namely HCV and HIV/AIDS (cf. Chapter 5). To date, HIV/AIDS has been the
BBVI responsible for the largest number of illicit drug-related deaths, and it is
likely that we will see a significant increase in deaths related to chronic HCV
infection in coming years, as cohorts of IDU with HCV infection age (Jager
et al., 2004; Lauer & Walker, 2001; Law et al., 2003).

Preventing the spread of infection through effective harm reduction interventions with IDU is the most effective way to reduce mortality related to these
infections. This might be achieved through: (a) reducing high-risk behaviour
among IDU; (b) the provision of sterile injecting equipment to IDU, or education about effective methods of decontaminating used injection equipment; (c)
availability of HIV and HCV testing for IDU; and (d) the provision of effective
drug treatments.

Education about the risks of HCV and HIV transmission through risk behaviours such as sharing injecting equipment and engaging in unprotected sex (in
the case of HIV) is indicated for IDU. The provision of testing for HIV and
HCV also enables users who have been diagnosed with the illness to access
treatment should they wish to receive it, and ensure they engage in safe injecting and sexual behaviours; such interventions have been argued to be of particular benefit for at risk groups such as IDU (Chou et al., 2005).

There is increasing evidence to suggest that needle and syringe programs
(NSPs), which provide sterile needles and syringes to IDU, reduce both drug
use and sexual risk behaviours of IDU (Cross et al., 1998; Gibson et al., 2001).
There is also evidence that they reduce the seroconversion rate of HIV among
this population, perhaps by as much as a third (Bastos & Strathdee, 2000;
Gibson et al., 2001; Hurley et al., 1997; Pollack & Heimer, 2004; Vlahov &
Junge, 1998).

The picture for HCV prevention is less positive, with agreement among
experts that NSPs are less effective in reducing the transmission of the disease
(Commonwealth Department of Health and Aging, 2002; Crofts et al., 2000).

In countries such as Australia where NSP provision has been thought to have successfully averted increased HIV infections among IDU, high rates of HCV infection still exist (Law et al., 2003). It is important to consider why this may be so. Two reasons are thought to explain this finding: first, the significantly higher infectivity of the HCV through blood to blood contact (Jager et al., 2004), and the higher baseline infection rate of HCV that is almost universally found amongst IDU (Jager et al., 2004).

As discussed above, there is good evidence that long-term drug treatment can reduce drug use, sharing of injecting equipment, antisocial behaviour, and other medical costs for opioid-dependent IDU. The reduced frequency of drug use and reduced risk behaviours suggests a reduced risk of contraction of HIV and HCV, which has been borne out by research, although the evidence for HIV prevention is much stronger (Ball et al., 1988; Metzger et al., 1998, 2000; Pollack & Heimer, 2004). One study examining HIV seroconversion rates found that clients who were in consistent MT were 6 times less likely than those out of treatment to seroconvert (Metzger et al., 1998). As noted for NSPs, there is less evidence that methadone maintenance is effective in reducing HCV transmission (Pollack & Heimer, 2004).

In summary, drug treatment and prevention interventions seem less effective for reducing HCV transmission because it is more easily transmitted than HIV and the base rate of infection is so much higher in IDU populations.

8.4.3 Suicide

As discussed in Chapter 7, suicide is a major clinical issue for users of illicit drugs, and one that has not been given the specific attention that it deserves. It is important to re-emphasise that suicide is a separate issue from that of drug overdose, a behaviour with which it is sometimes conflated.

One of the major findings of drug treatment outcome studies is that treatment substantially reduces rates of depression, as drug use and drug-related problems decline (Gossop et al., 2002a; Ward et al., 1998). As depression is a strong risk factor for suicide, suicide rates might also be expected to decline. The specific effects of treatment on suicide, rather than depression generally, have rarely been examined. A recent study, however, demonstrated that whilst treatment did indeed reduce rates of depression, rates of attempted suicide did not significantly decline (Darke et al., 2005e). Thus, drug treatment per se may not be sufficient. There are several reasons why this might be so. Whilst depression declines amongst a cohort, those with entrenched major depression may well not show reductions in depression and suicidal ideation. Also, a previous suicide attempt strongly predicts a subsequent one (Darke et al., 2005e; Gibbs et al., 2002). Finally, many suicide attempts are reactions to specific crises, which are beyond the scope of treatment to control. Drug use may well decline, but factors such as the threat of prison or a relationship break-up, may still trigger a suicide attempt.

Given the salience of depression and suicide as clinical factors, a specific clinical focus on these issues appears warranted. At the very least, regular screening amongst treatment populations for depression and suicidal ideation would help identify those at greatest risk. Specific intervention could be directed at those so identified. This may involve adjunct psychological interventions to reduce levels of depression and suicidal ideation and, possibly, the prescription of antidepressants. If the latter course is followed, it would appear that the use of tricyclics is strongly contraindicated. Amongst opioid users, these have been associated with fatal and non-fatal overdose (cf. Chapter 5). The cardiotoxic nature of these drugs also mitigates against their use with users of cocaine or amphetamine, given the cardiotoxic effects of these drugs. Selective serotonin re-uptake inhibitors (SSRIs) would appear a safer choice. The regular monitoring and management of life crises likely to increase suicide risk is also warranted. Being aware of impending court cases or relationship break-ups may appear prosaic, but in many cases it is such factors that precipitate a suicide attempt.

Suicide is an issue that has rarely been a subject of specific treatment intervention within the drug setting. The data suggest, however, that it is a major clinical issue in its own right, and is worthy of specific treatment resources. More specifically, it is an issue that would appear to be a high research priority. Major research priorities include the efficacy of screening for suicide risk within the treatment setting with appropriate referral, the provision of adjunct psychological counselling for suicidal ideation within the drug treatment setting, and the provision of SSRIs to those deemed at risk.

8.4.4   Trauma

As discussed in the previous chapter, the three main causes of traumatic death relevant to illicit drug users are motor vehicle accidents (MVAs), other forms of accident (e.g. drowning, falling from height), and homicide. Of these causes, the one that appears most amenable to being addressed is MVA. This is a major public health issue, and one that at least provides a specific behaviour that can be targeted, and evaluated by research. The major means of attempting to do so, clearly, would be interventions to reduce the frequency of drug intoxicated driving and consequent accidents. From an educational perspective, changing perceptions regarding drug driving amongst those who do drive under the influence of illicit drugs may well be beneficial. Drug drivers regard their behaviours as less dangerous than do others (Albery et al., 2000; Darke et al., 2003a; Kelly et al., 2004), because they mistakenly believe that they can still drive effectively, and not have accidents. The fact that they *cannot* drive as effectively, and *do* have a substantially higher risk of having accidents is clearly a message to be brought home. Research indicates that drug drivers are not deliberate "thrill seekers" and drive for quite prosaic reasons (Darke et al., 2003a). They may be potentially convinced to cease such behaviours. The use of roadside drug testing by police, an analogue to breath testing for alcohol, may be a more direct incentive to reduce the frequency of such behaviours (Jones et al., 2005). The efficacy of such interventions is clearly a high priority for research.

Unlike MVA trauma, non-MVA traumas do not provide a specific behavioural targets for intervention. These intoxicated accidents occur due to a range of causes, such falling from heights or drowning whilst intoxicated. Given the substantial role drugs play in such deaths, they do constitute a real public health issue. As with all public health issues, raising public awareness of the extent of the problem is necessary. Campaigns emphasising just how many accidental deaths are due to drug intoxication would be a useful beginning. How this would affect the behaviours of an intoxicated person is uncertain. As with the provision of overdose risk information, trials on the efficacy of such campaigns would appear warranted. To date, no such research has occurred, a reflection of the low salience of the issue generally. More specific interventions could clearly be focussed within workplaces involving high risks, such as factories. In such industries, arguments could be made for testing employees for *current* drug intoxication as a means of reducing risk.

It would appear that the only possible means of reducing the high rates of death by homicide amongst illicit drug users is by reductions in the drug use per se. It is drug use, drug seeking, and drug dealing that are likely to expose the individual to heightened risk of death by homicide. Drug treatment would appear to be the only realistic intervention to reduce such risks. To date, there are no data on the extent to which drug treatment reduces homicide rates amongst illicit drug users. Given the role homicide plays amongst these populations, such research is clearly important.

The paucity of research into traumatic death amongst illicit drug users was noted in Chapter 7. Apart from specific intervention research discussed above, general research into the contribution of trauma to drug-related mortality appears essential. Unlike areas such as HIV/AIDS, there is currently very little data upon which to base appropriate interventions.

8.5   Primary prevention

Considerable research and public interest has been focused upon ways in which substance use among young people may be reduced. The concept of "primary prevention" (or "demand reduction") can be applied in a number of ways, and the shape that prevention activities may take can also vary. Some interventions may target the whole population, on a school- or community-wide level. At the community level, drug awareness campaigns modelled upon social marketing principles are a politically popular option. Social marketing refers to a method used to achieve desirable behavioural change at the community level, typically involving mass marketing techniques that are used to correct misperceptions and to increase the social acceptability of a behaviour (Goren, 2005; Kotler & Zaltman, 1971). These techniques are commonly used tools for health promotion efforts that aim to influence social norms. Educational campaigns may be broadly targeted at the whole community, or towards particular subgroups such as drug users.

The use of "fear appeals" is common in social marketing practice (Hastings et al., 2004), particularly in the areas of alcohol and drug prevention (Goren, 2005). However, the evidence for the effectiveness of such approaches is far from satisfactory (Hastings et al., 2004). Some have responded to evidence of drug problems by developing education campaigns based upon promoting the risks in an emotive and dramatic fashion. Such responses reflect real concern by these groups, but they are probably ineffective in reducing harms related to the drug. This is because fear-based campaigns probably act in a divisive manner, with confirmed non-users having more negative views towards those who choose to use the drug, while the messages are most likely discounted by users who may view the material as exaggerating the risks.

One of most commonly implemented responses to concerns about drug use involves drug education with young people (McBride, 2003; Tobler & Stratton, 1997; White & Pitts, 1998). One meta-analytic review identified 595 different school-based drug education programs in Canada and the US alone (Tobler & Stratton, 1997). There is evidence to suggest that drug education may have a significant effect at the aggregate level in reducing self-reported drug use among young people at school (McBride, 2003; Tobler & Stratton, 1997; White & Pitts, 1998). The extent to which this translates into reduced mortality is unknown, but it is likely that such programs have less impact upon "at risk" youth, who may require more intensive interventions.

A range of interventions have been examined that target at risk youth, or which aim to address the risk factors for drug use and other outcomes such as school achievement and suicidal behaviours (National Research Council and Institute of Medicine, 2000; Vimpani, 2005). A comprehensive school-based programme designed to improve school bonding and reduce experiences of victimisation, the Victorian Gatehouse project (Patton et al., 2003), found evidence of reduced initiation of tobacco, alcohol, and cannabis use (Bond et al., 2004). There is also evidence that family-based interventions have a significant primary prevention effect for early onset alcohol use and intoxication (Foxcroft et al., 2003). Despite limited methodologically rigorous studies examining illicit drug use outcomes, a recent review concluded there was a strong suggestion that family involvement (with activities such as parenting skills, parental education about drugs, and skills increasing parents' confidence in communicating with young people about drugs) were important in preventing substance use among young people (Velleman et al., 2005; Vimpani, 2005). A consistent view of those reviewing the evidence in this area, however, has been that more carefully conducted evaluations of such interventions need to occur.

It is important to note that activities such as supply reduction may also have the consequence of reducing initiation to use of that drug (i.e. a primary prevention effect) (Day et al., in press-a; Degenhardt et al., 2005d; Ogilvie et al., 2005). This will be discussed further below.

8.6 Supply reduction

There has been much debate about the usefulness of supply reduction as a goal of drug policy. Before examining the evidence regarding the effectiveness of supply reduction it is useful to make clear what is meant by the term, as many often use the term as synonymous with street level drug law enforcement. "Supply reduction" refers to any policy aimed at reducing drug supply. It is not merely aimed at reducing *illicit* drug supply; many drug policies are aimed at reducing the supply of *licit* drugs such as alcohol or tobacco, and at drugs that are being used for recreational purposes rather than their desired function (e.g. nitrous oxide or petrol).

8.6.1 Legislative controls

Supply reduction policies in many cases refer to legislative controls. The case of licit drugs is one example, and there is good evidence to suggest that controlling supply through legislation that prohibits the manufacture, sale, and use of drugs is effective in reducing use and problems related to these drugs. There is also evidence to suggest that increasing the price of tobacco and alcohol through taxes is effective in reducing consumption at a population level (Hopkins et al., 2001; Ogilvie et al., 2005). Reducing availability through measures such as reduced operating hours for alcohol outlets, and controlling the number of outlets where cigarettes or alcohol may be sold are also effective in reducing the extent of use and harms related to these drugs (Norstrom & Skog, 2003; Ogilvie et al., 2005; Room et al., 2005). Changing the minimum legal drinking age for alcohol also has an effect: controlled studies in a number of countries have shown that raising the minimum legal drinking age reduces alcohol consumption and alcohol-related road crashes among young people (Ogilvie et al., 2005; Room et al., 2005). Similar interventions have also been targeted in communities experiencing problems related to substances such as petrol. Interventions in indigenous communities in Australia have shown a reduction in mortality related to petrol sniffing following the substitution of leaded petrol with unleaded petrol or Avgas (aviation fuel) (MacLean & D'Abbs, 2002).

In the case of illicit drugs, many of the legislative efforts involve legislation designed to reduce the availability of precursors. There is evidence to suggest that reducing the legal availability of precursors is associated with reduced harms related to the drugs produced from those precursors (Cunningham & Liu, 2005). Reductions in mortality might also be expected if this is taken to imply a reduction in the extent of use of such drugs.

8.6.2   Law enforcement

Supply reduction efforts also, of course, include drug law enforcement. It is important to make a distinction between lower-level (or "street level") policing, and higher-level law enforcement operations. Higher-level law enforcement activities may involve efforts to reduce drug production in source countries, efforts to reduce drug importation into destination countries, and operations targeting higher-level drug producers or traffickers. The extent to which these different higher-level intervention strategies are successful is determined in many ways by the multitude of factors affecting drug markets. What works in one context may well be inappropriate (or indeed counterproductive) in another.

8.6.2.1   Local level policing

There is consistent evidence suggesting that street level policing targeted at drug markets is not effective in reducing drug-related harm, but may even *increase* harms. The primary effect of street level policing appears to be in reducing the prominence of street level drug markets, and possibly improving public amenity (Edmunds et al., 1996; Graycar et al., 1999). There is less evidence that it is effective in reducing availability and purity, or increasing the price of drugs (Best et al., 2001; Dixon & Coffin, 1999), with some suggestion that displacement of drug sales to other locations will occur.

Studies conducted in a number of countries including the US, Canada, Australia, and the UK have consistently suggested that street level policing in areas where concentrated illicit drug markets exist is *not* effective in reducing drug use among users in that area (Aitken et al., 2002; Dixon & Coffin, 1999; Kerr et al., 2005; Maher & Dixon, 1999, 2001; May & Hough, 2001). There is also evidence that it increases risky behaviours such as sharing of injecting equipment, public injecting, and injecting a greater amount of drugs (Aitken et al., 2002; Cooper et al., 2005; Kerr et al., 2005; Maher & Dixon, 1999, 2001; May & Hough, 2001). All of these outcomes place users at greater risk of contracting BBVI and of overdosing.

8.6.2.2 High-level law enforcement

There is a dearth of empirical data on the effectiveness of high-level drug law enforcement (Manski et al., 2001), and a rarity of studies of the effects of abrupt changes in illicit drug supply in the world literature. There is considerable scepticism about the effectiveness of policies such as crop eradication and alternative crop development programs in countries growing coca and opium crops (Johnson, 2003; Kuo & Strathdee, 2005; Manski et al., 2001). In many instances, the consequences of crop eradication are most felt by poor farmers who are completely dependent upon the cash income from such crops to subsist. In many cases, crop eradication simply means greater debt is incurred by the farmers, who buy more seeds to replant them. In other instances, such as South American countries producing coca crops, there have been devastating effects of aerial crop spraying, which has often extended to the food crops farmers were also growing.

What happens if illicit drug supply is reduced? The Australian heroin shortage, which began early 2001 (Day et al., in press-b), has been the subject of considerable interest. Although there have been other major reductions in drug supply (Courtwright, 1982, 1990; Jonnes, 1996; Massing, 2000) these have been notable for their rarity. The Australian heroin shortage was probably due to a confluence of factors that reflected the complexity of the heroin market. One factor was probably the increased success of high-level Australian drug law enforcement operations conducted nationally and internationally

(Degenhardt et al., 2005f). These operations removed key individuals directing highly centralised drug trafficking networks that had supplied heroin to Australia, and resulted in the seizure of over 1000 kg of heroin in 2000 (Degenhardt et al., 2005f). Changes in source countries (e.g. reduced heroin production) may have played some role, but was not sufficient to explain the abrupt and sustained reduction in heroin supply in Australia. This was because other countries that sourced heroin from these same regions did not report any comparable abrupt reduction in heroin supply concurrently with, or after, the Australian shortage.

One of the most striking consequences of the heroin shortage in Australia was the significant decreases in non-fatal and fatal heroin overdoses (Degenhardt et al., 2005c, e). HCV notifications also decreased (Day et al., 2005), whereas mathematical models of the epidemic had predicted an increase (Law et al., 2003), an occurrence that may have been due to a reduction in the extent of injecting drug use in major markets (Day et al., 2004). Street drug markets also reduced in size, and drug sales became much less overt (Degenhardt et al., 2005b).

However, the reduction in heroin supply did have a number of other consequences. There were consistent reports that low- and mid-level heroin dealers shifted to dealing other drugs when heroin was less available to them (Degenhardt et al., 2005b). This finding was consistent with research examining changes in behaviour among low-level cannabis dealers when cannabis became less available (Loxley, 1998). There was also good evidence that users switched to using other drug types, including cocaine, methamphetamine, and injected benzodiazepines (Degenhardt et al., 2005e; Maher, 2002; Roxburgh et al., 2004; Topp et al., 2003).

It is important to consider whether the results of the work on the heroin shortage suggest that drug supply reduction should be a major focus of drug policy. There are reasons why it is necessary to be cautious about such simplistic statements. This event is obviously more relevant to countries in which heroin is a problem. Even in the case of heroin markets, it is necessary to be cautious because some of the reason for the reduction in heroin supply was possibly a fortunate coincidence of events. Further, this is most relevant to illicit drugs sourced from other countries. Countries with domestically sourced illicit drugs could not draw many policy conclusions from this event.

Achieving a relative reduction in drug supply in itself is not a sufficient policy response. The heroin shortage did not affect all heroin users in the same way (Degenhardt et al., 2005a, b, c; Degenhardt & Day, 2004; Maher, 2002). More disadvantaged-dependent heroin users shifted to riskier patterns of injecting drug use, experiencing substantial harm.

Australia has an integrated illicit drug policy that includes harm and demand reduction measures, such as increasing treatment places for opioid dependence and widespread availability of NSPs. The benefits of the reduction in heroin supply in Australia, therefore, occurred against a background of harm and demand reduction initiatives that probably reduced the severity of some of the negative consequences of reduced heroin supply. The benefits of the heroin shortage were, therefore, also due in part to concomitant harm reduction measures. It was clear from the work conducted on this event that both demand and harm reduction measures are required for users who continue to use drugs, despite a reduction in the supply of one particular drug.

8.7 Summary

Treatment for drug dependence substantially reduces rates of drug use, drug-related risk behaviours, and mortality, and will probably provide the most effective means to reduce illicit drug-related mortality. Treatment for two of the major causes of death amongst illicit drug users (HCV and HIV) has improved substantially in recent years, with the availability of new drug regimes. In addition to treatment interventions, a range of harm reduction measures have been implemented, or suggested, to reduce death from overdose or disease. These include targeted education on overdose, providing naloxone to opioid users, encouraging transitions in administration routes, medically supervised injecting centres, and the provision of sterile injecting equipment.

Suicide is a major cause of death among illicit drug users which is relatively unrecognised. Regular screening for depression and suicidal ideation may reduce suicide rates amongst illicit drug users. Death due to trauma may be more difficult to intervene against. The most feasible target would appear to be reductions in the frequency of drug-intoxicated driving.

Prevention and supply reduction are also components of multi-pronged approaches to reducing mortality. Positive family involvement appears to play an important role in preventing substance abuse among young people, and school-based programmes may also reduce the initiation drugs. There is limited evidence on the efficacy of law enforcement in reducing mortality. The recent Australian heroin shortage, however, may have been due in part to high-level law enforcement, and was associated with substantial decreases in heroin overdose and HCV notifications.

Key points: Summary of efforts to reduce illicit drug use-related mortality

- Treatment for drug dependence substantially reduces rates of drug use, drug-related risk behaviours and mortality.
- Recent years have seen significant developments in the treatment of HCV. Similarly, HAART has reduced deaths related to HIV/AIDS.
- Targeted education on overdose may reduce rates of morbidity and mortality. More controversial proposals include the provision of naloxone, encouraging transitions in routes of administration, and medically supervised injecting centres.
- There is increasing evidence that NSPs reduce seroconversion rates of HIV among IDU.
- Given that suicide is a major cause of death among illicit drug users, regular screening for depression, suicidal ideation, and likely trigger events appears warranted.
- The most feasible target for reducing traumatic death among illicit drug users is to reduce the frequency of drug-intoxicated driving.
- Positive family involvement appears to play an important role in preventing substance abuse among young people. There is also evidence that school-based programmes may also reduce the initiation of tobacco, alcohol and cannabis.
- There is limited evidence on the efficacy of law enforcement in reducing mortality. The recent heroin shortage seen in Australia, however, may have been due in part of high-level law enforcement, and was associated with substantial reductions in both heroin overdoses and HCV notifications.

9

Summary and conclusions

9.1 Introduction

Over the course of this book, we have examined many aspects of a particularly complex problem. In this chapter, we summarise the major findings from each of the areas covered and, briefly, look to the future.

9.2 Why should society care about drug-related death?

The question posed early in this book was: Does drug-related death matter? While it is undeniable that drug use and drug-related mortality have increased, should this be seen as a significant concern for society? As we saw, arguments could be made that these deaths are self-inflicted, and may even be of benefit to society due to reductions in crime and disease (Chapter 1). If we exclude simple compassion, which not all in a society would share, can the allocation of attention and resources to this problem be justified?

As was seen, the argument that death due to illicit drug use is an essentially self-inflicted harm does not stand up to any close intellectual scrutiny. Drug dependence is not an act of free will made in the absence of precipitating causes. There are a number of well-delineated psychosocial factors that engender dependent illicit drug use, most particularly the clinical picture of a "shattered childhood". Furthermore, and most importantly, we have seen that the majority of drug-related fatalities occur amongst drug-dependent individuals. These are people who have, by definition, lost control of their drug use. To have lost control of a problem clearly contradicts any arguments surrounding freely chosen lifestyles.

It is unarguable that illicit drug use imposes substantial costs upon society, through crime, disease, and lost years of productivity. As we have seen, however, drug users do not necessarily remain drug users. Drug treatment programmes have repeatedly been shown to make substantial impacts upon levels of drug use, crime, and health. There is also a well-delineated natural history to drug use, typically commencing in the teenage years, peaking in the 20s, and declining markedly after 30 years. Many, perhaps most, illicit drug users move beyond drug use to make substantial contributions to society. Finally, we must bear in mind the impact of drug-related death upon the families of decedents, and increases in the risks of "shattered childhoods" for the children of deceased users. Overall, there are cogent reasons why societies should care about drug-related death, that extend far beyond basic compassion.

9.3 How large is the problem?

It is one thing to care, but how big a problem are we to care about? Estimating the global mortality attributable to illicit drug use is no easy matter (Chapter 3). At least part of the difficulty is due to the very nature of the problem in question. Illicit drug use, by its very nature, involves people who conceal their drug use, and links between death and illicit drug use may not be recognised. While this will be less so for overdose, problems arise when estimating the role of suicide, disease, and trauma among illicit drug users. Even if we ignore this fundamental problem, the quality of official statistics on the prevalence of illicit drug-related mortality varies enormously from country to country. In particular, poorer nations simply do not have the resources to devote to data collection on these issues. Similarly, the extent of drug treatment and disease prevention programmes varies substantially from country to country, a fact that matters given that we have seen how much these programme impact upon drug use, disease, and mortality.

There are other limitations but, even so, some attempt must be made to estimate the size of the problem. Bearing these caveats in mind, it was estimated that approximately 200,000 deaths occurred worldwide in a single year (2000) that were attributable to illicit drug use (Degenhardt et al., 2004a). Importantly, and consistent with the rise in illicit drug use seen around the world, these deaths occurred in all world regions. The problem is clearly not the preserve of any one society, or group of societies. The majority of these cases are male, with an average age of around 30 years at death. The highest risk was seen to be associated with opioid use. The young profile of these deaths meant that they accounted for nearly 7 million disability adjusted life years (DALYs) in 2000 alone. The extent of the problem is further illustrated by longitudinal studies showing that illicit drug users die at rates more than 10 times those of their non-drug using peers.

Illicit drug use is a major cause of mortality worldwide, and involves substantial excess loss of life, and of potential productivity, particularly among the young. Moreover, this is a truly international problem, and not simply restricted to any one region.

9.4 What are the major causes of death?

What then are the main causes of such large, and elevated, death rates? As we have seen, these fall into the four broad areas of overdose (Chapter 4), disease (Chapter 5), suicide (Chapter 6), and trauma (Chapter 7).

Overdose is a major cause of death for users of opiates and cocaine. To a lesser extent it is also a mortality risk for amphetamine and 3,4-methylene-dioxymethamphetamine (MDMA) users. Given the increasing popularity of amphetamine and MDMA, the fact that they can, and do, cause death is an important finding documented in this book. There are, however, important differences between different drug classes in the mechanisms of overdose. While opioid overdose is primarily due to respiratory depression, cocaine and amphetamine toxicity relates more to myocardial infarction or stroke, and MDMA to the complications of hyperthermia. There are many issues, however, surrounding overdose that remain a mystery. Contrary to popular perception, it is not the young and inexperienced user who is the greatest overdose risk, but the long-term user. Why this is the case remains a matter of contention. Probably the most important finding in recent years from overdose research, however, has been the role of polydrug use. Single drug overdoses are rare, with the majority involving drug combinations. Alcohol, in particular, appears to play a major role in overdose deaths across a number of drug classes, albeit for different reasons. Understanding the role of multiple drug use in overdose points towards new measures to reduce such risk factors (cf. Chapter 8).

The second major cause of drug-related death is disease. Clearly, as distinct from overdose, disease is a cause of death relevant to both drug users and to non-drug users (Chapter 5). Illicit drug use, however, presents a range of disease risks either absent or present at much lower levels, amongst the general population. Large proportions of deaths amongst drug users are due to disease, and occur at rates many times those of non-drug users. The most salient are the blood-borne viruses (human immunodeficiency virus (HIV), hepatitis C virus (HCV), and hepatitis B virus (HBV)) transmitted through injecting with used injecting equipment and/or unprotected sexual activity. The impact of HIV infection in particular is enormous, accounting for the majority of disease-related deaths in many studies (cf. Chapter 5). We must bear in mind, however, that the role of disease in drug-related death is not restricted solely to transmissible diseases. As emphasised in earlier chapters, there are also specific pathologies that relate to the use of individual drugs. Cocaine and, to a lesser extent, amphetamine are cardiotoxic, and strongly associated with cardiovascular disease. We must also bear in mind the significant health effects of cannabis due to smoking as a route of administration.

The third major cause of death reviewed in this book was suicide (Chapter 6). Generally, when drug-related death is discussed, it is overdose and disease that come immediately to mind. We have seen, however, that suicide is a major killer of dependent drug users. Rates of completed, and attempted, suicide are many times higher than those of non-drug using peers, and suicide accounts for approximately one in ten drug user deaths. In fact, the proportion of drug users who attempt suicide in a single year is similar to the lifetime rate of the general population. While not given the attention it deserves, suicide is a major clinical problem among drug users, and a substantial challenge to those treating this group.

It is not surprising that suicide presents as such a significant cause of death, as dependent drug users typically present with an overwhelming range of risk factors. The shattered childhood of many of these users again comes to mind. Indeed, the known risk factors for suicide almost provide a redescription of the drug-dependent population.

Finally, it has been demonstrated that trauma accounts for a significant component of illicit drug user deaths (Chapter 7). Like suicide, this is an area that is under-explored. Regular illicit drug use, and dependent opiate and cocaine use in particular, is a risky business. Our review of the literature clearly showed that life-threatening events, and serious physical assault in particular, are common amongst illicit drug users, and occur at levels far higher than amongst their non-drug using peers. As we would expect, given such levels of exposure, mortality rates amongst illicit drug users due to trauma far exceed those of the general population. While the link between drug use and motor vehicle accident (MVA) is well recognised, the extent of excess death rates due to non-MVA trauma, such as drowning and homicide, are less well recognised. The dependent illicit drug user is at far greater risk of dying from drowning, or of being murdered, than are non-drug users. These issues are rarely discussed when looking at the clinical issues surrounding illicit drug use, but clearly contribute substantially to the elevated death rates seen among drug users.

9.5   What can we do to reduce death rates?

A brief summary of the clinical issues relating to drug-related mortality that are relevant to drug treatment, and other service, providers is presented in Table 9.1.

Table 9.1. Summary of clinical issues relating to the reduction of drug-related mortality for drug treatment and other agencies dealing with illicit drug users

Issue	Comment	Relevant chapters
Treatment	Long-term stable treatment reduces drug use and associated mortality	3, 8
Overdose		4, 8
• Education on risk factors		
Polydrug use	Education on risk of opioid and central nervous system drug use, cocaine, and alcohol use	
Cardiovascular disease	Education on psychostimulant toxicity risks from cardiovascular disease	
Dehydration/hyperthermia	Education for MDMA users	
• Improved response at overdose	Cardiopulmonary resuscitation training for users. Liaise with police to improve drug user emergency calls	
• Prison release	Emphasis on reduced tolerance if resume use	
• End of abstinent treatment	Emphasis on reduced tolerance if resume use	
• Naloxone provision	If legally possible, preliminary evidence suggests may improve responses at opioid overdose	
• Age	Emphasis on older drug users, who are most at risk	
Disease		5, 8
• Education		
Blood-borne viruses	Education on transmission routes of blood-borne viruses	
Cardiovascular disease	Education on cardiovascular disease and psychostimulants	
• Injecting equipment	Provision of sterile injecting equipment	
• Serostatus	Regular testing for HIV, HCV, HBV	
Suicide		6, 8
• Routine screening	Screen for depression, suicidal ideation, and precipitating events (e.g. marriage break-ups)	
• Co-morbid depression	Referral for treatment of major depression. Psychological interventions. If antidepressants prescribed, avoid tricyclics	
Trauma		7, 8
• Motor vehicle accident education	Education on dangers of drug driving	

In all probability, stable retention in drug treatment programmes will remain by far the most effective, and politically acceptable, means to reduce drug-related death. It is not, however, a panacea that results in the immediate cessation of all drug use and drug-related problems. As we have seen, however, drug treatment studies from many different countries repeatedly demonstrate the effectiveness of long-term treatments in reducing rates of drug use, drug-related problems, and mortality (cf. Chapter 8). By definition, a successful treatment that results in the cessation or amelioration of drug use removes or substantially reduces the risk of overdose. It will also reduce the risk of traumatic death through reductions in drug-intoxicated MVA rates, and other intoxicated traumatic accidents. Treatment would also appear to be the only means to reduce the elevated homicide rates among dependent drug users. Moreover, treatment improves overall physical health, and reduces the risk of infection with blood-borne viruses. Reduction in the other major risk factor, suicide, may require more direct psychological intervention as an adjunct to drug treatment. Given the salience of suicide as a cause of death, such interventions appear well worth implementing and evaluating (cf. Chapter 8).

Not all drug users are in treatment, and many who are will continue to use drugs whilst enrolled. In Chapter 8, we examined a range of non-drug treatment interventions addressing specific causes of death. These include well established, and evaluated, public health interventions such as needle and syringe exchange programmes, aimed at reducing the risk of infection with blood-borne viruses. In many countries, this form of intervention has been operating since the advent of the HIV pandemic amongst injecting drug users (IDUs). Other forms of death associated with illicit drug use, however, have not been so widely or directly addressed. We have seen how important overdose is, for example, as a leading cause of death. Education on the risks of polydrug use, improvements in responses to overdose, and the provision of naloxone to heroin users, have all been sporadically attempted and evaluated. The major risk of overdose resides among those outside the treatment system. It is to these users that specific interventions need to be targeted, and formally evaluated as high clinical and research priorities. As regards risk of traumatic death, intoxicated driving provides a specific behaviour that can, and should, be targeted amongst illicit drug users. Non-MVA trauma also accounts for a significant number of drug-related deaths, and could also clearly form a focus of intervention. The role of trauma, and non-MVA trauma in particular, are very poorly researched, and should form a significant research priority. These all provide examples of how we cannot rely solely on treatment programmes to reduce drug-related death.

The above interventions are aimed at those who already use illicit drugs. Attempts to prevent the use of these drugs, however, will always form part of any integrated approach to the reduction of drug-related mortality. While the research evidence on the efficacy of individual prevention programmes is not extensive, positive family involvement appears to play an important part in preventing substance abuse among young people. In light of the role that shattered childhoods from dysfunctional families play in the aetiology of illicit drug use, it makes sense that there is a positive role for functional families that are able to communicate with young people about the harms of illicit drugs. How prevention strategies and campaigns in schools and the general community may be more forcefully targeted is clearly a matter of considerable clinical and research interest.

Finally, we must not neglect the role of law enforcement in reducing the supply, use, and associated harms of illicit drugs. Throughout the course of this book, by its very nature, the high worldwide rates of mortality seen amongst illicit drug users has been emphasised. We do not know, however, how many lives have been saved by the fact that such drugs *are* illicit, and thus in restricted supply and use. The case of opioids, the most dangerous of the illicit drugs in terms of mortality risk, is illustrative. More widespread use of these drugs results in more deaths, particularly from overdose. There is a mortality risk associated with their use, and the more who use, the more who will die. Conversely, the recent heroin shortage seen in Australia saw substantial decreases in heroin overdoses and HCV notifications, as the use of the drug declined. Like all aspects of illicit drug policy, however, law enforcement must be seen in terms of a comprehensive approach involving treatment, prevention, and the reduction of avoidable harms. There is no single magic bullet to reduce illicit drug use death rates, and reductions will always involve multiple foci of intervention.

9.6   What does the future hold?

We are not seers, and cannot prognosticate with sibylline certainty what the future will hold. What is important, however, is that we should not assume that the patterns of mortality seen at the current time will always be the case. New causes of death may arise, and existing ones may become less important. In fact, we have already seen such a major change over the course of the last two decades. If we had been writing a comprehensive review of mortality amongst illicit drug users prior to the mid- to late-1980s, the focus on disease would have been substantially less. The HIV pandemic, however, changed the epidemiology of drug-related death, as well as responses to reduce mortality. A new emphasis on the sharing of injecting equipment as a means of viral transmission, with accompanying public health programmes such as needle and syringe exchanges, altered the nature of the drug debate. Even this newly emerged pattern, however, has been in flux. Let us take Italy as an example, a nation with has long had a high HIV seroprevalence amongst its IDU (Davoli et al., 1997; Quaglio et al., 2001). Until 1991, overdose was the major cause of heroin-related death (Quaglio et al., 2001). Between 1992 and 1996, however, acquired immunodeficiency syndrome (AIDS) usurped overdose as the major cause of death. New generation antiviral medications (Ellis et al., 2003; Vlahov et al., 2005) meant that subsequent to this AIDS-related death rates declined, with the result that overdose was once again the major killer. Clearly, the situation can change rapidly, even over the course of a single decade.

Apart from HIV, the disease that has emerged in the past two decades that has major long-term implications for drug-related mortality is HCV. Chronic HCV infection may result in chronic hepatitis, gross fatty metamorphosis of the liver, fibrosing liver disease, cirrhosis, and tumours (Karch, 2002). Given the high rates of infection amongst IDUs, the long-term impact upon mortality patterns is likely to be substantial. Importantly, HCV-related deaths may range beyond those attributed solely to disease. Chronic liver disease, with reduced capacity to metabolise drugs, may mean that more overdoses occur amongst the HCV infected. As with HIV, however, there is some cause for hope. Advances in the treatment of HCV infection through drugs such as the pegylated interferons hold considerable hope (Manns et al., 2001; Poynard, 2004). Again, the situation may change rapidly, and the relative contribution of disease to death may alter within a relatively brief period.

Drug use patterns, and thus the mortality resulting from such use, will always be in flux. At the beginning of this book, we noted the substantial increases in drug use and drug-related problems in countries such as China, India, and the republics of the former Soviet Union (Degenhardt et al., 2004a; United Nations Office for Drug Control, 2005). In these cases, new drug markets have emerged, and drug-related deaths have followed as a result. As emphasised earlier, illicit drug-related mortality is not the province of any one region or culture. Higher levels of international transport and integration suggest that the internationalisation of the problem is unlikely to reverse in the foreseeable future.

In addition to geographical changes in mortality patterns, we must also consider changes in patterns of drug use per se. These may be long-term shifts, or sudden, unexpected shifts. In Australia, in 2001, there was a sudden, unexpected, and prolonged reduction in the supply of heroin, an event so unusual that it attracted considerable international attention (Degenhardt et al., 2005e). As a result, heroin-related death declined significantly (Degenhardt et al., 2005c, e). The use of cocaine and more powerful forms of amphetamines, however, increased, as did the number of cocaine-related deaths seen at this time (Darke et al., 2005a; Degenhardt et al., 2005e; Topp et al., 2003). Clearly, the emphasis in overdose prevention in such a situation will have to change from a predominant emphasis on opioids to increased attention to psychostimulants. Indeed, internationally the continuing increase in the popularity of cocaine, amphetamine, and MDMA may change the profile of overdose deaths, and appropriate interventions. Chronic heart disease, for example, may play a far more significant role in international drug-related death than if opiates continue to dominate.

Finally, we must consider the effects that new cohorts of drug users will have on mortality. As we noted earlier (Chapter 3), in recent years the age of initiation to both licit and illicit drug use appears to be declining (Degenhardt et al., 2000; Mills et al., 2004). If such a trend were to continue, higher levels of drug dependence and more serious drug-related problems may well emerge (Fergusson & Horwood, 1997; Grant & Dawson, 1998; Mills et al., 2004). Given that earlier drug use onset is associated with a swifter and more severe problem development, we could expect rising death rates, occurring amongst even younger people than currently seen. As noted in Chapter 3, such a trend has already been noted in some jurisdictions (Hall et al., 1999a).

There are too many "ifs" and "buts" to make any comprehensive predictions on future mortality. What if all nations improved access to treatment, a known means of reducing mortality? What if they do the opposite? What if new diseases emerge? What if new drugs emerge? We cannot know. What we do know, however, is that change is the only certainty. We must accept this, and constantly monitor drug use patterns and related problems. Otherwise, we run the risk of constantly fighting the previous war.

9.7   Concluding remarks

To conclude, it can be seen that mortality amongst illicit drug users is a complex, over-determined problem. Death comes early for many such users in many forms, and at rates far higher than if they were not drug users. The four major causes of death (overdose, disease, suicide, trauma) each present specific problems for intervention. Can we reduce the level of mortality we currently see? Clearly, the answer is yes. We must not be too negative, as much progress has been made over the past few decades, and much more can be achieved from what we currently know. Treatment, in particular, is the most effective means of reducing mortality. Increasing access to, and enrolment in, drug treatment programmes is a high priority. The provision of new drug dependence treatments is a clear step in the right direction. A range of other interventions could be expanded, or trialled. We are now much better informed regarding the risk factors for drug overdose among different drug classes. Increasing such awareness of risk factors among the drug users themselves is crucial, as is improving their responses at overdoses. The early data on naloxone provision to reduce opioid overdose death rates are encouraging, and suggest that formal trials should be conducted. While controversial in many jurisdictions, the provision of sterile injecting equipment is a well established and evaluated intervention, and provides a front line intervention against blood-borne infections that appears worthy of continued implementation. We certainly could improve the provision of well-documented treatments for depression within the drug treatment setting, as a means to reduce the high suicide rates of drug users.

Much has been achieved, but if we were giving a school report card on our efforts to date it would have to read *could do better*. Indeed, from the perspective of the cost to society, *must do better* would provide a better imperative. We do not pretend to provide the answer to the numerous problems that surround drug use mortality. The first step, as always, is to understand the nature of the problem, stripped of preconceptions. Then, and only then, can we improve our efforts across the myriad problems that we are faced with.

References

Abdul-Quader, A.S., Friedman, S.R., Des Jarlais, D., Marmor, M.M., Maslansky, R. & Bartelme, S. (1987) Methadone maintenance and behavior by intravenous drug users that can transmit HIV. *Contemporary Drug Problems, 14*, 425–434.

Aceijas, C., Stimson, G., Hickman, M. & Rhodes, T. (2004) Global overview of injecting drug use and HIV infection among injecting drug users. *AIDS, 18*, 2295–2303.

Aderjan, R., Hoemann, S., Schmitt, G. & Skopp, G. (1995) Morphine and morphine glucuronides in serum of heroin consumers and in heroin-related deaths determined by HPLC with native fluorescence detection. *Journal of Analytical Toxicology, 19*, 163–168.

Agar, M. (2003) The story of crack: towards a theory of illicit drug trends. *Addiction Research and Theory, 11*, 3–29.

Aitken, C., Kerger, M. & Crofts, N. (2000) Drivers who use illicit drugs: behaviour and perceived risks. *Drugs: Education, Prevention and Policy, 7*, 39–50.

Aitken, C., Moore, D., Higgs, P., Kelsall, J. & Kerger, M. (2002) The impact of a police crackdown on a street scene: evidence from the street. *International Journal of Drug Policy, 13*, 193–200.

Albertson, T.E., Derlet, R.W., Van Hoozen, B.E. (1999) Methamphetamine and the expanding complications of amphetamines. *The Western Journal of Medicine, 170*, 214–219.

Albery, I., Gossop, M., Strang, J. & Griffiths, P. (2000) Illicit drugs and driving: prevalence, beliefs and accident involvement among a cohort of current out-of-treatment drug users. *Drug and Alcohol Dependence, 58*, 197–204.

Allison, M., Hubbard, R.L. & Ginzburg, H.M. (1985) Indicators of suicide and depression among drug abusers. 1979–1981 TOPS Admission Cohorts. *National Institute on Drug Abuse Treatment Monograph Series*. Rockville, MD US Department of Health and Human Services.

Altman, J., Everitt, B., Glautier, S., Markou, A., Nutt, D., Oretti, R., Phillips, G. & Robbins, T. (1996) The biological, social and clinical bases of drug addiction: commentary and debate. *Psychopharmacology, 125*, 285–345.

Amato, L., Davoli, M., Perucci, C.A., Ferri, M., Faggiano, F. & Mattick, R.P. (2005) An overview of systematic reviews of the effectiveness of opiate maintenance therapies: available evidence to inform clinical practice and research. *Journal of Substance Abuse Treatment, 28,* 321–329.

American Psychiatric Association (2000) *Diagnostic and Statistical Manual of Mental Disorders* (4th ed. Text Revision). Washington, DC: American Psychiatric Association.

Andreasson, S. & Allebeck, P. (1990) Cannabis and mortality among young men: a longitudinal study of Swedish conscripts. *Scandinavian Journal of Social Medicine, 18,* 9–15.

Anthony, J.C. & Helzer, J. (1991) Syndromes of drug abuse and dependence. In L.N. Robins & D.A. Regier (Eds), *Psychiatric disorders in America* (pp. 116–154). New York: The Free Press.

Anthony, J.C., Warner, L. & Kessler, R. (1994) Comparative epidemiology of dependence on tobacco, alcohol, controlled substances, and inhalants: basic findings from the National Comorbidity Survey. *Experimental and Clinical Psychopharmacology, 2,* 244–268.

Appleby, L., Cooper, J., Amos, T. & Faragher, B. (1999) Psychological autopsy study of suicides by people under 35. *British Journal of Psychiatry, 175,* 168–174.

Ashton, C.H. (1999) Adverse effects of cannabis and cannabinoids. *British Journal of Anaesthesia, 83,* 637–649.

Athanaselis, S., Dona, A., Papadodima, S., Papoutsis, G., Maravelias, C. & Koutselinis, A. (1999) The use of alcohol and other psychoactive substances by victims of traffic accidents in Greece. *Forensic Science International, 102,* 103–109.

Australian Bureau of Statistics (2004) *Year Book Australia 2003.* Canberra: Australian Bureau of Statistics.

Australian Institute of Health and Welfare (2005) *2004 National Drug Strategy Household Survey: First results.* Canberra: Australian Institute of Health and Welfare.

Bachman, J.G., Wadsworth, K.N., O'Malley, P., Johnston, L. & Schulenberg, J. (1997) *Smoking, drinking and drug use in young adulthood: the impacts of new freedoms and responsibilities.* Mahwah, NJ: Lawrence Erlbaum.

Baddour, L.M., Meyer, J. & Henry, B. (1991) Polymicrobial infective endocarditis in the 1980s. *Reviews of Infectious Diseases, 13,* 963–970.

Ball, J.C., Lange, W., Myers, C. & Friedman, S.R. (1988) Reducing the risk of AIDS through methadone maintenance treatment. *Journal of Health and Social Behavior, 29,* 214–226.

Ball, J.C. & Ross, A. (1991) *The effectiveness of methadone maintenance treatment: Patients, programs, services, and outcome.* Vienna: Springer-Verlag.

Bargagli, A.M., Sperati, A., Davoli, F., Forastiere, F. & Perucci, C.A. (2001) Mortality among problem drug users in Rome: an 18-year follow-up study, 1980–1997. *Addiction, 96,* 1455–1463.

Bartu, A., Freeman, N.C., Gawthorne, G.S., Codde, J.P. & Holman, D.J. (2004) Mortality in a cohort of opiate and amphetamine users in Perth, Western Australia. *Addiction, 99,* 60–63.

Bastos, F.I. & Strathdee, S. (2000) Evaluating effectiveness of syringe exchange programmes: current issues and future prospects. *Social Science and Medicine*, *51*, 1771–1782.

Beautrais, A.L., Joyce, P.R., Mulder, R.T., Fergusson, D.M., Deavoll, B.J. & Nightingale, S.K. (1996) Prevalence and comorbidity of mental disorders in persons making serious suicide attempts: a case–control study. *American Journal of Psychiatry*, *153*, 1009–1014.

Beck, A.T., Steer, R.A., Kovacs, M. & Garrison, B. (1985) Hopelessness and eventual suicide: a 10-year prospective study of patients hospitalized with suicidal ideation. *American Journal of Psychiatry*, *142*, 559–563.

Benhamou, Y., Bochet, M., Di Martino, V., Charlotte, F., Azria, F. & Coutellier, A. (1999) Liver fibrosis progression in human immunodeficiency virus and hepatitis C virus coinfected patients. *Hepatology*, *30*, 1054–1058.

Bennett, G. & Higgins, D. (1999) Accidental overdose among injecting drug users in Dorset, UK. *Addiction*, *94*, 1179–1190.

Benson, G. & Holmberg, M.B. (1984) Drug-related mortality in young people. *Acta Pyschiatrica Scandinavia*, *70*, 525–534.

Bentley, A.J. & Busuttil, A. (1996) Deaths among drug abusers in south-east Scotland (1989–1994). *Medicine Science and the Law*, *36*, 231–236.

Best, D., Gossop, M., Man, L., Finch, E., Greenwood, J. & Strang, J. (2000) Accidental and deliberate overdose among opiate addicts in methadone maintenance treatment: are deliberate overdoses systematically different? *Drug and Alcohol Review*, *19*, 213–216.

Best, D., Strang, J., Beswick, T. & Gossop, M. (2001) Assessment of a concentrated, high-profile police operation: no discernible impact on drug availability, price or purity. *British Journal of Criminology*, *41*, 738–745.

Bewley, T.H., Ben-Arie, O. & James, I.P. (1968) Morbidity and mortality from heroin dependence. 1: survey of heroin addicts known to the home office. *British Medical Journal*, *1*, 725–732.

Beyrer, C., Jittiwutikarn, J., Teokul, W., Razak, M.H., Suriyanon, V., Srirak, N., Vongchuk, T., Tovanabutra, S., Sripaipan, T. & Celentano, D.D. (2003) Drug use, increasing incarceration rates, and prison-associated HIV risks in Thailand. *AIDS and Behavior*, *7*, 153–161.

Blix, O. & Grönbladh, L. (1988) AIDS and IV heroin addicts: The preventive effect of methadone maintenance in Sweden. Paper presented to *Fourth International Conference on AIDS*, Stockholm, Sweden.

(1991) The impact of methadone maintenance on the spread of HIV among IV drug users in Sweden. In N. Loimer, R. Schmid & A. Springer (Eds), *Drug addiction and AIDS* (pp. 200–205). Vienna: Springer-Verlag.

Blomberg, R. & Preusser, D. (1974) Narcotic use and driving behaviour. *Accident Analysis and Prevention*, *6*, 23–32.

Blows, S., Ivers, R., Connors, J., Ameratunga, S., Woodward, M. & Norton, R. (2005) Marijuana use and car crash injury. *Addiction*, *100*, 605–611.

Bobashev, G.V. & Anthony, J.C. (1998) Clusters of marijuana use in the United States. *American Journal of Epidemiology*, *148*, 1168–1174.

Bond, L., Patton, G., Glover, S., Carlin, J., Butler, H., Thomas, L. & Bowes, G. (2004) The Gatehouse Project: can a multilevel school intervention affect emotional well-being and health risk behaviours? *Journal of Epidemiology and Community Health*, *58*, 997–1003.

Borges, G., Walters, E.E. & Kessler, R.C. (2000) Associations of substance use, abuse, and dependence with subsequent suicidal behaviour. *American Journal of Epidemiology*, *151*, 781–789.

Borgia, G., Reynaud, L., Gentile, I. & Piazza, M. (2003) HIV and hepatitis C virus: facts and controversies. *Infection*, *31*, 232–240.

Bowling, B. (1999) The rise and fall of New York murder: zero tolerance or crack's decline? *British Journal of Criminology*, *39*, 531–554.

Boyd, J., Randell, T., Luurila, H. & Kuisma, M. (2003) Serious overdoses involving buprenorphine in Helsinki. *Acta Anaestiologica Scandinavia*, *47*, 1031–1033.

Bradley, R.H. & Corwyn, R.F. (2002) Socioeconomic status and child development. *Annual Review of Psychology*, *53*, 371–399.

Broers, B., Junet, C., Bourquin, M., Deglon, J.J., Perrin, L. & Hirschel, B. (1998) Prevalence and incidence rate of HIV, hepatitis B and C among drug users on methadone maintenance treatment in Geneva between 1988 and 1995. *Aids*, *12*, 2059–2066.

Brook, J.S., Whiteman, M., Gordon, A. & Brook, D. (1988) The role of older brothers in younger brothers' drug use viewed in the context of parent and peer influences. *Journal of Genetic Psychology*, *151*, 59–75.

Brookoff, D., Rotondo, M.F., Shaw, L.M., Campbell, E.A. & Fields, L. (1996) Cocaethylene levels in patients who test positive for cocaine. *Annals of Emergency Medicine*, *27*, 316–320.

Brosnich, T. & Wittchen, H.U. (1994) Suicidal ideation and suicide attempts: comorbidity with depression, anxiety disorders, and substance use disorder. *European Archives of Clinical Neuroscience*, *244*, 93–98.

Brown, L.S., Chu, A., Nemoto, T., Ajuluchukwu, D. & Primm, B.J. (1989) Human immunodeficiency virus infection in a cohort of intravenous drug users in New York City: demographic, behavioral, and clinical features. *New York State Journal of Medicine*, *89*, 506–510.

Brugal, M.T., Domingo-Salvany, A., Puig, R., Barrio, G., Garcia de Olalla, P. & de la Fuente, L. (2005) Evaluating the impact of methadone maintenance programmes on mortality due to overdose and AIDS in a cohort of heroin users in Spain. *Addiction*, *100*, 981–989.

Bryant, W.K., Galea, S., Tracy, M., Piper, T.M., Tardiff, K.J. & Vlahov, D. (2003) Overdose deaths attributed to methadone and heroin in New York City, 1990–1998. *Addiction*, *99*, 846–854.

Bucknall, A.B.V. & Robertson, J.R. (1986) Deaths of heroin users in a general practice. *Journal of the Royal College of General Practitioners*, *36*, 120–122.

Buckstein, O.G., Brent, D.A., Perper, J.A., Moritz, G., Baugher, M., Schweers, J., Roth, C. & Balach, L. (1993) Risk factors for suicide among adolescents with a history of substance use: a case-control study. *Acta Psychiatrica Scandinavia*, *88*, 403–408.

Budd, J., Copeland, L., Elton, R. & Robertson, R. (2002) Hepatitis C infection in a cohort of injecting drug users: past and present risk factors and the implications for educational and clinical management. *European Journal of General Practice*, *8*, 95–100.

Bull, S.S., Piper, P. & Rietmeijer, C. (2002) Men who have sex with men and also inject drugs–profiles of risk related to the synergy of sex and drug injection behaviors. *Journal of Homosexuality*, *42*, 31–51.

Burns, J.M., Martyres, R.F., Clode, D. & Boldero, J.M. (2004) Overdose in young people using heroin: associations with mental health, prescription drug use and personal circumstances. *Medical Journal of Australia*, *181*, S25–S28.

Buster, M.C.A., van Brussel, G.H.A. & van den Brink, W. (2002) An increase in overdose mortality during the first 2 weeks after entering or re-entering methadone treatments in Amsterdam. *Addiction*, *97*, 993–1001.

Busto, U.E., Kaplan H.L., Wright C.E., Gomez-Mancilla B., Zawertailo L., Greenblatt D.J. & Sellers E.M. (2000) A comparative pharmacokinetic and dynamic evaluation of alprazolam sustained-release, bromazepam, and lorazepam. *Journal of Clinical Psychopharmacology*, *20*, 628–635.

Bux, D., Lamb, R. & Iguchi, M. (1995) Cocaine use and HIV risk behaviour in methadone maintenance patients. *Drug and Alcohol Dependence*, *37*, 29–35.

Cami, J., Farre, M., Mas, M., Roset, P., Poudevida, S., Mas, A., San, L. & de la Torre R. (2000) Human pharmacology of 3, 4-methylenedioxymeth-amphetamine ("Ecstasy"): psychomotor performance and subjective effects. *Journal of Clinical Psychopharmacology*, *20*, 455–466.

Canetto, S.S. & Sakinofsky, I. (1998) The gender paradox in suicide. *Suicide and Life-Threatening Behavior*, *28*, 1–23.

Cantor, C., McTaggart, P. & Deleo, D. (2001) Misclassification of suicide-the contribution of opiates. *Psychopathology*, *34*, 140–145.

Caplehorn, J.R.M. (1996) Risk factors for non-HIV-related death among methadone maintenance patients. *European Addiction Research*, *2*, 49–52.

Caplehorn, J. R. M., Dalton, M.S.Y.N., Cluff, M.C. & Petrenas, A.M. (1994) Retention in methadone maintenance and heroin addicts' risk of death. *Addiction*, *89*, 203–207.

Caplehorn, J.R.M., Dalton, M.S., Haldar, F., Petrenas, A. & Nisbet, J.G. (1996) Methadone maintenance addicts' risk of fatal heroin overdose. *Substance Use and Misuse*, *31*, 177–196.

Carpenter, M.J., Chutuape, M.A. & Stitzer, M.L. (1998) Heroin snorters versus injectors: comparison on drug use and treatment outcome in age-matched samples. *Drug and Alcohol Dependence*, *53*, 11–15.

Carrel, T., Schaffner, A., Vogt, P., Laske, A., Niederhauser, U., Schneider, J. & Turina, M. (1993) Endocarditis in intravenous drug addicts and HIV infected patients: possibilities and limitations of surgical treatment. *Journal of Heart Valve Disease*, 2, 140–147.

Carrieri, M.P., Rey, D., Loundou, A., Lepeu, G., Sobel, A., Obadia, Y. and the MANIF-2000 Study Group (2003) Evaluation of buprenorphine maintenance in a French cohort of HIV-infected injecting drug users. *Drug and Alcohol Dependence*, 72, 13–21.

Casey, P.R. (1989) Personality disorder and suicide intent. *Acta Psychiatrica Scandinavia*, 79, 290–295.

Casado, J.L., Sabido, R., Perez-Elias, M.J., Antela, A., Oliva, J., Dronda, F., Mejia, B. & Fortun, J. (1999) Percentage of adherence correlates with the risk of protease inhibitor (PI) treatment failure in HIV-infected patients. *Antiviral Therapy*, 4, 157–161.

Castilla, J., Del Romero, J., Hernando, V., Marincovich, B., Garcia, S. & Rodriguez, C. (2005) Effectiveness of highly active antiretroviral therapy in reducing heterosexual transmission of HIV. *Journal of Acquired Immune Deficiency Syndromes*, 40, 96–101.

Centers for Disease Control (2003) Deaths, percent of total deaths, and death rates for the 15 leading causes of death in selected age groups by race and sex: United States 2000. Atlanta: Centers for Disease Control.

Chaisson, R.E., Bacchetti, P., Osmond, D., Brodie, B., Sande, M.A. & Moss, A.R. (1989) Cocaine use and HIV infection in intravenous drug users in San Francisco. *JAMA*, 261, 561–565.

Chatham, L.R., Knight, K., Joe, G.W. & Simpson, D.D. (1995) Suicidality in a sample of methadone maintenance patients. *American Journal of Drug and Alcohol Abuse*, 21, 345–361.

Chen, K. & Kandel, D.B. (1995) The natural history of drug use from adolescence to the mid-thirties in a general population sample. *American Journal of Public Health*, 85, 41–47.

Cherubin, C., McCusker, J., Baden, M., Kavaler, F. & Amsel, Z. (1972) The epidemiology of death in narcotic addicts. *American Journal of Epidemiology*, 96, 11–22.

Cherubin, C.E. & Sapira, J.D. (1993) The medical complications of drug addiction and the medical assessment of the intravenous drug user: 25 years later. *Annals of Internal Medicine*, 119, 1017–1028.

Chesney, M., Morin, M. & Sherr, L. (2000) Adherence to HIV combination therapy. *Social Science and Medicine*, 50, 1599–1605.

Chesher, G. & Hall, W. (1999) Effects of cannabis on the cardiovascular and gastrointestinal systems. In H. Kalant, W. Corrigall, W. Hall & R. Smart (Eds), *The health effects of cannabis* (pp. 435–458). Toronto, Ont.: Centre for Addiction and Mental Health.

Chiasson, M., Stoneburner, R., Hildebrandt, D., Ewing, W., Telzak, E. & Jaffe, H. (1991) Heterosexual transmission of HIV-1 associated with the use of smokable freebase cocaine (crack) *AIDS*, 5, 1121–1126.

Chou, R., Huffman, L., Fu, R., Smits, A. & Korthuis, T. (2005) Screening for HIV: a review of the evidence for the US preventive services task force. *Annals of Internal Medicine, 143*, 55–73.

Cicchetti, D. & Rogosch, F.A. (1999) Psychopathology as risk for adolescent substance use disorders: a developmental psychopathology perspective. *Journal of Clinical Child Psychology, 28*, 355–365.

Clark, H.W., Masson, C.L., Delucchi, K.L., Hall, S.M. & Sees, K.L. (2001) Violent traumatic events and drug abuse severity. *Journal of Substance Abuse Treatment, 20*, 121–127.

Coffin, P.O., Galea, S., Ahern, J., Leon, A.C., Vlahov, D. & Tardiff, K. (2003) Opiate, cocaine and alcohol combinations in accidental drug overdose deaths in New York City, 1990–1998. *Addiction, 98*, 739–747.

Commonwealth Department of Health and Aging (2002) *Return on investment in needle and syringe exchange programs in Australia.* Canberra: Commonwealth Department of Health and Aging.

Coomber, R. (1997) How often does the adulteration/dilution of heroin actually occur? An analysis of 228 "street" heroin samples across the UK (1995–96) and discussion of monitoring policy. *International Journal of Drug Policy, 8*, 178–186.

(1999) The cutting of heroin in the United States in the 1990s. *Journal of Drug Issues, 29*, 17–36.

Cooncool, B., Smith, H. & Stimmel, B. (1979) Mortality rates of persons entering methadone maintenance: a seven-year study. *American Journal of Drug and Alcohol Abuse, 6*, 345–353.

Cooper, H., Moore, L.D., Gruskin, S. & Krieger, N. (2005) The impact of a police crackdown on drug injectors' ability to practice harm reduction: a qualitative study. *Social Science and Medicine, 61*, 673–684.

Cooper-Patrick, L., Crum, R. & Ford, D.E. (1994) Identifying suicidal ideation patients in general medical practice. *JAMA, 272*, 1757–1762.

Copeland, A.R. (1984) Deaths during recreational activity. *Forensic Science International, 25*, 117–122.

Copeland, J. & Dillon, P. (2005) The health and psychosocial consequences of ketamine use. *International Journal of Drug Policy, 16*, 122–131.

Costa, G.M., Pizzi, C., Bresciani, B., Tumscitz, C., Gentile, M. & Bugiardini, R. (2001) Acute myocardial infarction caused by amphetamines: a case report and review of the literature. *Italian Heart Journal, 2*, 478–480.

Costello, E., Erkanli, A., Federman, E. & Angold, A. (1999) Development of psychiatric comorbidity with substance abuse in adolescents: effects of timing and sex. *Journal of Clinical Child Psychology, 28*, 298–311.

Cottler, L.B., Compson, W.M., Mager, D., Spitznagel, E.L. & Janca, A. (1992) Posttraumatic stress disorder among substance abusers from the general population. *American Journal of Psychiatry, 149*, 664–670.

Cottrell, D., Childs-Clarke, A. & Ghodse, A.H. (1985) British opiate addicts: an 11-year follow-up. *British Journal of Psychiatry, 146*, 448–450.

Courtwright, D. (1982) *Dark Paradise: Opiate Addiction in America before 1940.* Cambridge, MA: Harvard University Press.

Courtwright, D., Joseph, H. & Des Jarlais, D. (1990) *Addicts Who Survived: An Oral History of Narcotic Addiction in America 1923–1965.* Knoxville, TN: University of Tennessee.

Crofts, N., Hopper, J.L., Bowden, D., Breschkin, A.M., Milner, R. & Locarnini, S. A. (1993) Hepatitis C virus infection among a cohort of Victorian injecting drug users. *Medical Journal of Australia, 159,* 237–241.

Crofts, N., Stewart, T., Hearne, P., Ping, X.Y., Breschkin, A.M. & Locarnini, S.A. (1995) Spread of bloodborne viruses among Australian prison entrants. *British Medical Journal, 310,* 285–288.

Crofts, N., Aitken, C. & Kaldor, J. (1999) The force of numbers: why hepatitis C is spreading among Australian injecting drug users while HIV is not. *Medical Journal of Australia, 170,* 220–221.

Crofts, N., Caruana, S., Bowden, S. & Kerger, M. (2000) Minimising harm from hepatitis C virus needs better strategies. *British Medical Journal, 321,* 899.

Cross, J.C., Saunders, C. & Bartelli, D. (1998) The effectiveness of educational and needle exchange programs: a meta-analysis of HIV prevention strategies for injecting drug users. *Quality and Quantity, 32,* 165–180.

Cunningham, J. & Liu, M.L. (2005) Impacts of federal precursor chemical regulations on methamphetamine arrests. *Addiction, 100,* 479–488.

Darke, S. & Hall, W. (1995) Levels and correlates of polydrug use among heroin users and regular amphetamine users. *Drug and Alcohol Dependence, 39,* 231–235.

(1997) The distribution of naloxone to heroin users. *Addiction, 92,* 1195–1199.

(2003) Heroin overdose: research and evidence-based intervention. *Journal of Urban Health: Bulletin of the New York Academy of Medicine, 80,* 189–200.

Darke, S. & Kaye, S. (2004) Attempted suicide among injecting and non-injecting cocaine users in Sydney, Australia. *Journal of Urban Health: Bulletin of the New York Academy of Medicine, 81,* 505–515.

Darke, S. & Ross, J. (1997a) Polydrug dependence and psychiatric comorbidity among heroin injectors. *Drug and Alcohol Dependence, 48,* 135–141.

(1997b) Overdose risk perceptions and behaviours among heroin users in Sydney, Australia. *European Addiction Research, 3,* 87–92.

(2000a) The use of antidepressants among injecting drug users in Sydney, Australia. *Addiction, 95,* 407–417.

(2000b) Fatal heroin overdoses resulting from non-injecting routes of administration, NSW, Australia, 1992–1996. *Addiction, 95,* 596–599.

(2001) The relationship between suicide and overdose among methadone maintenance patients in Sydney, Australia. *Addiction, 96,* 1443–1453.

(2002) Suicide among heroin users: rates, risk factors and methods. *Addiction, 97,* 1383–1394.

Darke, S. & Zador, D. (1996) Fatal heroin overdose: a review. *Addiction, 91,* 1765–1772.

Darke, S., Cohen, J., Ross, J., Hando, J. & Hall, W. (1994) Transitions between routes of administration of regular amphetamine users. *Addiction*, *89*, 1077–1083.

(1995) Injecting and sexual risk-taking behaviour among regular amphetamine users. *AIDS Care*, *7*, 19–26.

(1996a) Overdose among heroin users in Sydney, Australia I. Prevalence and correlates of non-fatal overdose. *Addiction*, *91*, 405–411.

(1996b) Overdose among heroin users in Sydney, Australia II. Responses to overdose. *Addiction*, *91*, 413–417.

Darke, S., Sunjic, S., Zador, D. & Prolov, T. (1997) A comparison of blood toxicology of heroin-related deaths and current heroin users in Sydney, Australia. *Drug and Alcohol Dependence*, *47*, 45–53.

Darke, S., Kaye, S. & Finlay-Jones, R. (1998) Antisocial personality disorder, psychopathy and injecting drug use. *Drug and Alcohol Dependence*, *52*, 63–69.

Darke, S., Hall, W., Weatherburn, D. & Lind, B. (1999) Fluctuations in heroin purity and the incidence of fatal heroin overdose. *Drug and Alcohol Dependence*, *54*, 155–161.

Darke, S., Ross, J., Zador, D. & Sunjic, S. (2000) Heroin-related deaths in New South Wales, Australia, 1992–1996. *Drug and Alcohol Dependence*, *60*, 141–150.

Darke, S., Kaye, S. & Ross, J. (2001) Geographical injecting locations among injecting drug users in Sydney, Australia. *Addiction*, *96*, 241–246.

Darke, S., Hall, W., Kaye, S., Ross, J. & Duflou, J. (2002) Hair morphine concentrations of fatal heroin overdose cases and living heroin users. *Addiction*, *97*, 977–984.

Darke, S., Kelly, E. & Ross, J. (2003a) Drug use and driving among injecting drug users in Sydney, Australia: prevalence, risk factors and risk perceptions. *Addiction*, *99*, 175–185.

Darke, S., Mattick, R. & Degenhardt, L. (2003b) The ratio of non-fatal to fatal overdose. *Addiction*, *98*, 1169–1170.

Darke, S., Ross, J. & Lynskey, M. (2003c) The relationship of conduct disorder to attempted suicide and drug use history among methadone maintenance patients. *Drug and Alcohol Review*, *22*, 21–25.

Darke, S., Ross, J., Lynskey, M. & Teesson, M. (2004) Attempted suicide among entrants to three treatment modalities for heroin dependence in the Australian Treatment Outcome Study (ATOS): prevalence and risk factors. *Drug and Alcohol Dependence*, *73*, 1–10.

Darke, S., Kaye, S. & Duflou, J. (2005a) Cocaine-related fatalities in New South Wales, Australia 1993–2002. *Drug Alcohol Dependence*, *77*, 107–114.

Darke, S., Ross, J., Teesson, M. (2005b) Twelve month outcomes for heroin dependence treatments: does route of administration matter? *Drug and Alcohol Review*, *24*, 165–171.

Darke, S., Ross, J., Teesson, M., Ali, R., Cooke, R., Ritter, A. & Lynskey, M. (2005c) Factors associated with 12 months continuous heroin abstinence: findings from the Australian Treatment Outcome Study (ATOS). *Journal of Substance Abuse Treatment*, *28*, 255–263.

Darke, S., Ross, J., Williamson, A. & Teesson, M. (2005d) The impact of borderline personality disorder on 12 month outcomes for the treatment of heroin dependence. *Addiction*, *100*, 1121–1130.

(2005e) Attempted suicide among heroin users: 12 month outcomes from the Australian Treatment Outcome Study (ATOS). *Drug and Alcohol Dependence*, *78*, 177–186.

(2005f) Heroin overdose, treatment exposure and client characteristics: findings from the Australian Treatment Outcome Study (ATOS). *Drug and Alcohol Review*, *24*, 425–432.

Davidson, P.J., McLean, R.L., Kral, A.H., Gleghorn, A.A., Edlin, B.R. & Moss, A.R. (2003) Fatal heroin-related overdose in San Francisco, 1997–2000: a case for targeted intervention. *Journal of Urban Health: Bulletin of the New York Academy of Medicine*, *80*, 261–273.

Davis, G.G. & Swalwell, C.I. (1994) Acute aortic dissections and ruptured berry aneurysms associated with methamphetamine abuse. *Journal of Forensic Sciences*, *39*, 1481–1485.

Davoli, M., Perucci, C.A., Forastiere, F., Doyle, P., Rapiti, E., Zaccarelli, M. & Abenti, D.D. (1993) Risk factors for overdose mortality: a case control study within a cohort of intravenous drug users. *International Journal of Epidemiology*, *22*, 273–277.

Davoli, M., Perucci, C.A., Rapiti, E., Bargagli, A.M., Dippoliti, D., Forastiere, F. & Abeni, D. (1997) A persistent rise in mortality among injection drug users in Rome, 1980 through 1992. *American Journal of Public Health*, *87*, 851–853.

Day, C., Degenhardt, L., Gilmour, S. & Hall, W. (2004) Effects of a reduction in heroin supply on injecting drug use: analysis of data from needle and syringe programmes. *British Medical Journal*, *329*, 428–429.

(2005) Changes in blood-borne virus notifications and injecting related harms following reduced heroin supply in New South Wales, Australia. *BMC Public Health*, *5*(84).

Day, C., Degenhardt, L. & Hall, W. (in press-a) Changes in the initiation of heroin use after a reduction in heroin supply. *Drug and Alcohol Review*. Day, C., Degenhardt, L. & Hall, W. (in press-b) NSW heroin markets: Documenting the heroin shortage. *Drug and Alcohol Review*.

Degenhardt, L. & Day, C. (Eds) (2004) *The course and consequences of the heroin shortage in New South Wales. NDLERF Monograph No. 4*. Adelaide: Australasian Centre for Policing Research.

Degenhardt, L., Lynskey, M. & Hall, W. (2000) Cohort trends in the age of initiation of drug use in Australia. *Australian and New Zealand Journal of Public Health*, *24*, 421–426.

Degenhardt, L., Hall, W. & Lynskey, M. (2001) The relationship between cannabis use, depression and anxiety among Australian adults: findings from the national survey of mental health and well-being. *Social Psychiatry and Psychiatric Epidemiology*, *36*, 219–227.

Degenhardt, L., Darke, S. & Dillon, P. (2003) The prevalence and correlates of GHB overdose among Australian users. *Addiction*, *98*, 199–204.

Degenhardt, L., Hall, W., Warner-Smith, M. & Lynskey, M. (2004a) Illicit drug use. In M. Ezzati, A. Lopez, A. Rodgers & C.J.L. Murray (Eds), *Comparative quantification of health risks. global and regional burden of disease Attributable to Selected Major Risk Factors*, Vol. 1 (pp 1111–1175). Geneva: World Health Organization.

Degenhardt, L., Rendle, V., Hall, W., Gilmour, S. & Law, M. (2004b) *Estimating the number of heroin users in NSW and Australia, 1997–2002. NDARC Technical Report No. 198.* Sydney: National Drug and Alcohol Research Centre, University of New South Wales.

Degenhardt, L., Conroy, E., Day, C., Gilmour, S. & Hall, W. (2005a) The impact of the Australian heroin shortage on demand for and compliance with treatment for drug dependence. *Drug and Alcohol Dependence*, *79*, 129–135.

Degenhardt, L., Conroy, E., Gilmour, S. & Collins, L. (2005b) The effect of a reduction in heroin supply in Australia upon drug distribution and acquisitive crime. *British Journal of Criminology*, *45*, 2–24.

Degenhardt, L., Conroy, E., Gilmour, S. & Hall, W. (2005c) The effect of a reduction in heroin supply upon population trends in fatal and non-fatal drug overdoses. *Medical Journal of Australia*, *182*, 20–23.

Degenhardt, L., Day, C., Conroy, E., Gilmour, S. & Hall, W. (2005d) Age differentials in the impacts of reduced heroin supply: effects of a "heroin shortage" in NSW, Australia. *Drug and Alcohol Dependence*, *79*, 397–404.

Degenhardt, L., Day, C., Dietze, P., Pointer, S., Conroy, E., Collins, L. & Hall, W. (2005e) Effects of a sustained heroin shortage in three Australian states. *Addiction*, *100*, 908–920.

Degenhardt, L., Reuter, P., Collins, L. & Hall, W. (2005f) Evaluating explanations of the Australian "heroin shortage". *Addiction*, *100*, 459–469.

Degenhardt, L., Roxburgh, A. & Barker, B. (2005g) Underlying causes of cocaine, amphetamine and opioid-related deaths in Australia. *Journal of Clinical Forensic Medicine*, *12*, 187–195.

Denning, D.G., Conwell, Y., King, D. & Cox, C. (2001) Method choice, intent and gender in completed suicide. *Suicide and Life-Threatening Behavior*, *30*, 282–288.

Department of Health and Human Services (2005) *Drug Abuse Warning Network, 2003: Area Profiles of Drug-related Mortality.* DAWN Series D-27. Rockville, MD: Department of Health and Human Services.

Derlet, R.W. & Horowitz, B.Z. (1995) Cardiotoxic drugs. *Emergency Medicine Clinics of North America*, *13*, 771–791.

Derlet, R.W., Rice, P., Horowitz, B.Z. & Lord, R.V. (1989) Amphetamine toxicity: experience with 127 cases. *The Journal of Emergency Medicine*, *7*, 157–161.

Des Jarlais, D.C., Friedman, S.R., Novick, D.M., Sotheran, J.L., Thomas, P., Yancovitz, S.R., et al. (1989) HIV-1 infection among intravenous drug users in Manhattan, New York City, from 1977 through 1987. *JAMA*, *261*, 1008–1012.

Desmond, D.P., Maddux, J.F. & Trevino, A. (1978) Street heroin potency and deaths from overdose in San Antonio. *American Journal of Drug and Alcohol Abuse*, *5*, 39–49.

Dettmer, K., Saunders, B. & Strang, J. (2001) Take home naloxone and the prevention of deaths from opiate overdose: two pilot schemes. *British Medical Journal*, *322*, 895–896.

Diekstra, R.F.W. & Gulbinat, W. (1993) The epidemiology of suicidal behaviour: a review of three continents. *World Health Statistics Quarterly*, *46*, 52–68.

Digiusto, E., Shakeshaft, A., Ritter, A., O'Brien, S., Mattick, R.P. & the NEPODResearch Group (2004) Serious adverse events in the Australian National Evaluation of Pharmacotherapies for Opioid Dependence (NEPOD). *Addiction*, *99*, 450–460.

Dinwiddie, S.H., Reich, T. & Cloninger, C.R. (1992) Psychiatric comorbidity and suicidality among intravenous drug users. *Journal of Clinical Psychiatry*, *53*, 364–369.

Dinwiddie, S.H., Cottler, L., Compton, W. & Abdallah, A.B. (1996) Psychopathology and HIV risk behaviours among injection drug users in and out of treatment. *Drug and Alcohol Dependence*, *43*, 1–11.

Dixon, D. & Coffin, P. (1999) Zero tolerance policing of illegal drug markets. *Drug and Alcohol Review*, *18*, 477–486.

Doherty, M.C., Garfein, R.S., Monterroso, E., Brown, D. & Vlahov, D. (2000) Correlates of HIV infection among young adult short-term injection drug users. *AIDS*, *14*, 717–726.

Dolan, K., Wodak, A., Hall, W., Gaughwin, M. & Rae, F. (1996) Risk behaviour of IDUs before, during and after imprisonment in NSW. *Addiction Research*, *4*, 151–160.

Dolan, K., Kimber, J., Fry, C., Fitzgerald, J., McDonald, D. & Trautmann, F. (2000) Drug consumption facilities in Europe and the establishment of supervised injecting centres in Australia. *Drug and Alcohol Review*, *9*, 337–346.

Dolan, K., Shearer, J., MacDonald, M., Mattick, R.P., Hall, W. & Wodak, A.D. (2003) A randomised controlled trial of methadone maintenance treatment versus wait list control in an Australian prison system. *Drug and Alcohol Dependence*, *72*, 59–65.

Dolan, K.A., Shearer, J., White, B., Zhou, J., Kaldor, J. & Wodak, A.D. (2005) Four-year follow-up of imprisoned male heroin users and methadone treatment: mortality, re-incarceration and hepatitis C infection. *Addiction*, *100*, 820–828.

Dole, V.P., Nyswander, M.E. & Kreek, M.J. (1966) Narcotic blockade. *Archives of Internal Medicine*, *118*, 304–309.

Drucker, E. (1999) Drug prohibition and public health: 25 years of evidence, *Public Health Reports*, *114*, 14–29.

Drummer, O., Gerostamoulos, J., Batziris, H., Chu, M., Caplehorn, J.R.M., Robertson, M.D. & Swann, P. (2003) The involvement of drugs in drivers of motor vehicles killed in Australian road traffic crashes. *Accident Analysis and Prevention*, *36*, 239–248.

Drummer, O.H., Syrjanen, M., Opeskin, K. & Cordner, S. (1990) Deaths of heroin addicts starting on a methadone maintenance programme. *Lancet*, *335*, 108.

Duburcq, A., Charpak, Y., Blin, P. & Madec, L. (2000) Two year follow-up of heroin users treated by GPs with higher dosage buprenorphine. *Revue Epidemiologie et de Sante Publique*, *48*, 363–373.

Drummer, O.H., Opeskin, K., Syrjanen, M. & Cordner, S.M. (1992) Methadone toxicity causing death in ten subjects starting on a methadone maintenance program. *American Journal of Forensic Medicine and Pathology, 13*, 346–350.

Duflou, J. & Mark, A. (2000) Aortic dissection after ingestion of "ecstasy" (MDMA). *The American Journal of Forensic Medicine and Pathology, 21*, 261–263.

Dukes, P.D., Robinson, G.M. & Robinson, B.J. (1992) Mortality of intravenous drug users: attenders of the Wellington drug clinic, 1972–1989. *Drug and Alcohol Review, 11*, 197–201.

Dziukas, L.J. & Vohra, J. (1991) Tricyclic antidepressant poisoning. *Medical Journal of Australia, 154*, 344–350.

Edlin, B., Irwin, K., Faraque, S., McCoy, C. & Word, C. (1994) Intersecting epidemics – crack cocaine use and HIV infection among inner city young adults. Multicenter Crack Cocaine and HIV Infection Study Team. *New England Journal of Medicine, 331*, 1422–1427.

Edmunds, M., Hough, M. & Urquia, N. (1996) *Tackling local drug markets. Crime detection and prevention series No. 80*. London: Home Office.

Edwards, G. & Gross, M. (1976) Alcohol dependence: provisional description of a clinical syndrome. *British Medical Journal, 1*, 1058–1061.

Edwards, G., Gross, M., Keller, M., Moser, J. & Room, R. (1977) *Alcohol-related disabilities*. Geneva: World Health Organization.

Ellinwood, E.H. & Nikaido, A.M. (1987) Stimulant induced impairment: a perspective across dose and duration of use. *Alcohol Drugs and Driving, 3*, 19–24.

Engstrom, A., Adamsson, C.M., Allebeck, P. & Rydberg, W. (1991) Mortality in patients with substance abuse: a follow-up in Stockholm County, 1973–1984, *International Journal of the Addictions, 26*, 91–106.

Ellis, R.J., Childers, M.E., Cherner, M., Lazzaretto, D., Letendre, S., Grant, I. & HIV Neurobehavioral Research Center Group (2003) Increased human immunodeficiency virus loads in active methamphetamine users are explained by reduced effectiveness of antiretroviral therapy. *Journal of Infectious Diseases, 188*, 1820–1826.

Eskild, A., Magnus, P., Samuelson, S.O., Soholberg, C. & Kittelsen, P. (1993) Differences in mortality rates and causes of death between HIV positive and HIV negative intravenous drug users. *International Journal of Epidemiology, 22*, 315–320.

Esteban, J., Gimeno, C., Barril, J., Aragones, A., Climent, J.M. & de al Cruz-Pellin, M. (2003) Survival study of opioid addicts in relation to its adherence to methadone maintenance treatment. *Drug and Alcohol Dependence, 70*, 193–200.

European Monitoring Centre for Drugs and Drug Addiction (1997) *Estimating the prevalence of problem drug use in Europe* (Scientific Monograph 1) Luxembourg: European Monitoring Centre for Drugs and Drug Addiction.

(1999a) *Literature Review on the Relation Between Drug Use, Impaired Driving and Traffic Accidents*. Lisbon: European Monitoring Centre for Drugs and Drug Addiction.

(1999b) *Study to Obtain Comparable National Estimates of Problem Drug Use Prevalence for all EU Member States*. Lisbon: European Monitoring Centre for Drugs and Drug Addiction.

(2004) *Annual Report on the State of Drugs in the European Union and Norway*. Lisbon: European Monitoring Centre for Drugs and Drug Addiction.

(2005) *Annual Report 2005: The state of the drugs problem in the European Union and Norway*. Lisbon: European Monitoring Centre for Drugs and Drug Addiction.

Ezzati, M. & Lopez, A. (2004) Smoking and oral tobacco use. In M. Ezzati, A. Lopez, A. Rodgers & C.J.L. Murray (Eds), *Comparative quantification of health risks. Global and regional burden of disease attributable to selected major risk factors*, Vol. 1 (pp 883–958). Geneva: World Health Organization.

Ezzati, M., Lopez, A., Rodgers, A. & Murray, C.J.L. (Eds) (2004) *Comparative Quantification of Health Risks. Global and Regional Burden of Disease Attributable to Selected Major Risk Factors*. Geneva: World Health Organization.

Farnsworth, T.L., Brugger, C.H. & Malters, P. (1997) Myocardial infarction after intranasal methamphetamine. *American Journal of Health-System Pharmacy*, *54*, 586–587.

Farrell, M., Marsden, J., Ali, R. & Ling, W. (2002) Methamphetamine: drug use and psychoses becomes a major public health issue in the Asia Pacific region. *Addiction*, *97*, 771–772.

Fergusson, D.M. & Lynskey, M.T. (1995) Childhood circumstances, adolescent adjustment, and suicide attempts in a New Zealand Birth Cohort. *Journal of the American Academy of Child and Adolescent Psychiatry*, *34*, 612–622.

Fergusson, D.M. & Horwood, L.J. (1997) Early onset cannabis use and psychosocial adjustment in young adults. *Addiction*, *92*, 279–296.

Fineschi, V. & Masti, A. (1996) Poisoning by MDMA (ecstasy) and MDEA: a case report. *International Journal of Legal Medicine*, *108*, 272–275.

Fischer, B., Kendall, P., Rehm, J. & Room, R. (1997) Charting WHO-goals for licit and illicit drugs for the year 2000: are we "on track"? *Public Health*, *111*, 271–275.

Frischer, M., Bloor, M., Goldberg, D., Clark, J., Green, S. & McKeganey, N. (1993) Mortality among injecting drug users: a critical reappraisal. *Journal of Epidemiology and Community Health*, *47*, 59–63.

Flynn, P.M., Joe, G.W., Broome, K.M., Simpson, D.D. & Brown, B.S. (2003) Recovery from opioid addiction in DATOS. *Journal of Substance Abuse Treatment*, *25*, 177–186.

Foxcroft, D., Ireland, D., Lister-Sharp, D., Lowe, G. & Breen, R. (2003) Longer-term primary prevention for alcohol misuse in young people: a systematic review. *Addiction*, *98*, 397–411.

Friedman, L.N., Williams, M.T., Singh, T.P. & Friedman, T.R. (1996) Tuberculosis, AIDS, and death among substance abusers on welfare in New York City. *New England Journal of Medicine*, *334*, 828–833.

Frischer, M., Goldberg, D., Rahman, M. & Berney, L. (1997) Mortality and survival among a cohort of drug injectors in Glasgow, 1982–1994. *Addiction*, *92*, 419–427.

Fukunaga, T., Mizoi, Y. & Adachi, J. (1987) Methamphetamine-induced changes of peripheral catecholamines: an animal experiment to elucidate the cause of sudden death after methamphetamine abuse. *Japanese Journal of Legal Medicine*, *41*, 335–341.

Fugelstad, A., Rajs, J., Bottiger, M., Gehrardsson, M. & de Verdier, M.G. (1995) Mortality among HIV-infected intravenous addicts in Stockholm in relation to methadone treatment. *Addiction*, *90*, 711–716.

Fugelstad, A., Annell, A., Rajs, J. & Angren, G. (1997) Mortality and causes and manner of death among drug addicts in Stockholm during the period 1981–1992. *Acta Pyschiatrica Scandinavia*, *96*, 169–175.

Fugelstad, A., Ahlner, J., Brandt, L., Ceder, G., Eksborg, S., Rajs, J. & Beck, O. (2003) Use of morphine and 6-monoacetylmorphine in blood for the evaluation of possible risk factors for sudden death in 192 heroin users. *Addiction*, *98*, 463–470.

Furst, S.R., Fallon, S.P., Reznik, G.N. & Shah, P.K. (1990) Myocardial infarction after inhalation of methamphetamine. *New England Journal of Medicine*, *323*, 1147–1148.

Gagajewski, A. & Apple, F.S. (2003) Methadone-related deaths in Hennepin County, Minnesota, 1992–2002. *Journal of Forensic Sciences*, *48*, 668–671.

Galea, S., Nandi, V.V. & Vlahov, D. (2004) The social epidemiology of substance use. *Epidemiologic Reviews*, *26*, 36–52.

Galea, S., Worthington, N., Piper, T.M., Nandi, V.V., Curtis, M. & Rosenthal, D.M. (2006) Provision of naloxone to injection drug users as an overdose prevention strategy: Early evidence from a pilot study in New York City. *Addictive Behaviors*, *31*, 907–912.

Galli, M. & Musicco, M. (1994) Mortality of intravenous drug users living in Milan, Italy: role of HIV-I infection. *AIDS*, *8*, 1457–1463.

Gardner, R. (1970) Deaths in United Kingdom opioid users, 1965–1968. *Lancet*, September 26, 650–653.

Garnefski, N. & Diekstra, R.F.W. (1997) Child sexual abuse and emotional and behavioural problems in adolescence: gender differences. *Journal of the American Academy of Child and Adolescent Psychiatry*, *36*, 323–329.

Garten, R.J., Lai, S., Zhang, J., Liu, W., Chen, J., Vlahov, D. & Yu, X.F. (2004) Rapid transmission of hepatitis C virus among young injecting heroin users in Southern China. *International Journal of Epidemiology*, *33*, 182–188.

Gayet-Ageron, A., Baratin, D., Marceillac, E., Allard, R., Peyramond, D., Chidiac, C., Trepo, C., Livrozet, J.M., Touraine, J.L., Ritter, J., Sepetjan, M., Fabry, J. & Vanhems, P. (2004) The AIDS epidemic in Lyon: patient characteristics and defining illnesses between 1985 and 2000. *HIV Medicine*, *5*, 163–170.

Gearing, F.R. & Schweitzer, M.D. (1974) An epidemiologic evaluation of long-term methadone maintenance treatment for heroin addiction. *American Journal of Epidemiology*, *100*, 101–112.

Gebo, K.A., Diener-West, M. & Moore, R.D. (2003) Hospitalization rates differ by hepatitis C status in an urban HIV cohort. *Journal of Acquired Immune Deficiency Syndromes*, *34*, 165–173.

Gerostamoulos, J., Staikos, V. & Drummer, O.H. (2001) Heroin-related deaths in Victoria: a review of cases for 1997 and 1998. *Drug and Alcohol Dependence*, *61*, 123–127.

Ghodse, H., Oyefesso, A. & Kilpatrick, B. (1998) Mortality of drug addicts in the United Kingdom 1967–1993. *International Journal of Epidemiology*, *27*, 473–478.

Gibbs, S.J., Beautrais, A.L. & Fergusson, D.M. (2005) Mortality and further suicidal behaviour after an index suicide attempt: a 10-year study. *Australian and New Zealand Journal of Psychiatry, 39*, 95–100.

Gibson, D., Flynn, N. & Perales, D. (2001) Effectiveness of syringe exchange programs in reducing HIV risk behaviour and HIV seroconversion among injecting drug users. *AIDS, 15*, 1329–1341.

Gill, J.R. (2001) Fatal descent from height in New York City. *Journal of Forensic Science, 46*, 1132–1137.

Gill, J.R. & Catanese, C. (2002) Sharp injury fatalities in New York City. *Journal of Forensic Sciences, 47*, 554–557.

Gill, J.R., Hayes, J.A., deSouza, I.S., Marker, E. & Stajic, M. (2002) Ecstasy (MDMA) Deaths in New York City: a case series and review of the literature. *Journal of Forensic Sciences, 47*, 121–126.

Gill, J.R., Lenz, K.A. & Amolat, M.J. (2003) Gunshot fatalities in children and adolescents in New York City. *Journal of Forensic Sciences, 48*, 832–835.

Gill, K., Nolimal, D. & Crowley, J. (1992) Antisocial personality disorder, HIV risk taking behaviour and retention in methadone maintenance therapy. *Drug and Alcohol Dependence, 30*, 247–252.

Gill, K. & Stajic, M. (2000) Ketamine in non-hospital and hospital deaths in New York City. *Journal of Forensic Sciences, 45*, 655–658.

Gittelman, R., Mannuzza, S., Shenker, R. & Bonagura, N. (1985) Hyperactive boys almost grown up: I. Psychiatric status. *Archives of General Psychiatry, 42*, 937–947.

Gjerde H., Beylich K.M. & Morland J. (1993) Incidence of alcohol and drugs in fatally injured car drivers in Norway. *Accident Analysis and Prevention, 25*, 479–483.

Global and Regional Burden of Disease Attributable to Selected Major Risk Factors. World Health Organization, Geneva.

Goedert, J.J., Pizza, G., Gritti, F.M., Costiogliola, P., Boschini, A., Bini, A., Lazzari, C. & Palareti, A. (1995) Mortality among drug users in the AIDS era. *International Journal of Epidemiology, 24*, 1204–1210.

Goldstein, A. & Herrara, J. (1995) Heroin addicts and methadone treatment in Albuquerque: a 22-year follow-up. *Drug and Alcohol Dependence, 40*, 139–150.

Goren, N. (2005) *Social marketing: prevention and practice review*. Melbourne: Centre for Youth Drug Studies, Australian Drug Foundation.

Gossop, M., Marsden, J., Stewart, D., Edwards, C., Lehmann, P., Wilson, A. & Segar, G. (1998) Substance use, health and social problems of service users at 54 drug treatment agencies: intake data from the national treatment outcome research study. *British Journal of Psychiatry, 193*, 166–171.

Gossop, M., Marsden, J., Stewart, D. & Rolfe, A. (1999) Treatment retention and 1 year outcomes for residential programmes in England. *Drug and Alcohol Dependence, 57*, 89–98.

(2000) Patterns of improvement after methadone treatment: 1 years follow-up results from the National Treatment Outcome Research Study. *Drug and Alcohol dependence*, *60*, 275–286.

Gossop, M., Marsden, J., Stewart, D. & Treacy, S. (2002a) Change and stability of change after treatment of drug misuse. 2 year outcomes from the National Treatment Outcome Research Study. *Addictive Behaviours*, *27*, 155–166.

Gossop, M., Steward, D., Treacy, S. & Marsden, J. (2002b) A prospective study of mortality among drug misusers during a four year period after seeking treatment. *Addiction*, *97*, 39–47.

Gourevitch, M.N. & Friedland, G.H. (2000) Interactions between methadone and medications used to treat HIV infection: a review. *Mount Sinai Journal of Medicine*, *67*, 429–436.

Gowing, L., Farrell, M., Bornemann, R. & Ali, R. (2004) Substitution treatment of injecting opioid users for prevention of HIV infection. *The Cochrane Database of Systematic Reviews.*

Gowing, L.R., Henry-Edwards, S.M., Irvine, R.J. & Ali, R.L. (2002) The health effects of ecstasy. *Drug and Alcohol Review*, *21*, 53–63.

Graham, H. & Power, C. (2004) Childhood disadvantage and health inequalities:a framework for policy based on lifecourse research. *Child Care: Health and Development*, *30*, 671–678.

Grant, B.F. & Dawson, D.A. (1998) Age of onset and its association with DSM-IV drug abuse and dependence: results form the National Longitudinal Alcohol Epidemiological Survey. *Journal of Substance Abuse*, *10*, 163–173.

Graycar, A., Nelson, D. & Palmer, M. (1999) *Law enforcement and illicit drug control. AIC trends and issues in crime and criminal justice bulletin No. 110*. Canberra: Australian Institute of Criminology.

Greenberg, M., Hamilton, R. & Toscano, G. (1999) Analysis of toxicology reports from the 1993–1994 census of fatal occupational injuries. *Compensation and Working Conditions*, *4*, 26–28.

Greenfield, S.F. & O'Leary, G. (1999) Sex differences in marijuana use in the United States. *Harvard Review of Psychiatry*, *6*, 297–303.

Grönbladh, L. & Gunne, L.M. (1989) Methadone-assisted rehabilitation of Swedish heroin addicts. *Drug and Alcohol Dependence*, *24*, 31–37.

Gronbladh, L., Ohland, L.S. & Gunne, L.M. (1990) Mortality in heroin addiction: impact of methadone treatment. *Acta Psychiatrica Scandinavia*, *82*, 223–227.

Guharoy, R., Medicis, J., Choi, S., Stalder, B., Kusiowski, K. & Allen, A. (1999). Methamphetamine overdose: experience with six cases. *Veterinary & Human Toxicology*, *41*, 28–30.

Gutierrez-Cebollada, J., De La Torre, R., Ortuno, J., Garces, J. & Cami, J. (1994) Psychotropic drug consumption and other factors associated with heroin overdose, *Drug and Alcohol Dependence*, *35*, 169–174.

Haarstrup, S. & Jepson, P.W. (1988) Eleven year follow-up of 300 young opioid addicts. *Acta Psychiatrica Scandinavia*, *77*, 22–26.

Hales, G., Roth, N. & Smith, D. (2000) Possible fatal interaction between protease inihibitors and methamphetamine. *Antiretroviral Therapies*, *5*, 19.

Halkitis, P., Parsons, J.T. & Stirratt, M. (2001) A double epidemic: crystal methamphetamine use in relation to HIV transmission among gay men. *Journal of Homosexuality*, *41*, 17–35.

Hall, W., Degenhardt, L. & Lynskey, M. (1999a) Opioid overdose mortality in Australia, 1964–1997: birth cohort trends. *Medical Journal of Australia*, *171*, 34–37.

Hall, W., Johnston, L. & Donnelly, N. (1999b) Epidemiology of cannabis use and its consequences. In H. Kalant, W. Corrigall, W. Hall & R. Smart (Eds), *The Health Effects of Cannabis* (pp. 71–125). Toronto, Ont.: Centre for Addiction and Mental Health.

Hall, W., Teesson, M., Lynskey, M. & Degenhardt, L. (1999c) The 12-month prevalence of substance use and ICD-10 substance use disorders in Australian adults: findings from the National Survey of Mental Health and Well-Being. *Addiction*, *94*, 1541–1550.

Hall, W., Lynskey, M. & Degenhardt, L. (2000) Trends in opiate-related deaths in the United Kingdom and Australia, 1985–1995, *Drug and Alcohol Dependence*, *57*, 247–254.

Hall, W., Degenhardt, L. & Lynskey, M. (2001) *The health and psychological consequences of cannabis use* (NCADA Monograph No. 44). Canberra: Australian Publishing Service.

Hardman, J.G., Limbird, L.E., Molinoff, P.B., Ruddon, R.W. & Gilman, A.G. (Eds) (1996) *Goodman & Gilman's The Pharmacological Basis of Therapeutics (9th edition)*. New York: McGraw-Hill.

Harlow, K.C. (1990) Patterns of rates of mortality from narcotics and cocaine overdose in Texas, 1976–1987. *Public Health Reports*, *105*, 455–462.

Harris, E.C. & Barraclough, B. (1997) Suicide as an outcome for mental disorders. *British Journal of Psychiatry*, *170*, 205–228.

(1998) Excess mortality of mental disorder. *British Journal of Psychiatry*, *173*, 11–53.

Harris, D.S., Everhart, E.T., Mendelson, J. & Jones, R.T. (2003) The pharmacology of cocaethylene in humans following cocaine and ethanol administration. *Drug and Alcohol Dependence*, *72*, 169–182.

Harruff, R.C., Francisco, J.T., Elkins, S.K., Phillips, A.M. & Fernandez, G.S. (1988) Cocaine and homicide in Memphis and Shelby County: an epidemic of violence. *Journal of Forensic Sciences*, *33*, 1231–1237.

Hartel, D.M., Schoenbaum, E.E., Selwyn, P.A., Friedland, G.H., Klein, R.S. & Drucker, E. (1996) Patterns of heroin, cocaine and speedball injection among methadone maintenance patients: 1978–1988. *Addiction Research*, *4*, 323–340.

Hartnoll, R. (1997) Cross-validating at local level. In European Monitoring Centre for Drugs and Drug Addiction (Ed.), *Estimating the prevalence of problem drug use in Europe* (pp. 247–261). Luxembourg: Office for Official Publications of the European Communities.

Hassan, R. (1995) *Suicide explained. The Australian experience.* Melbourne: Melbourne University Press.

Hastings, G., Stead, M. & Webb, J. (2004) Fear appeals in social marketing: strategic and ethical reasons for concern. *Psychology and Marketing, 21*, 961–986.

Hawkins, J., Catalano, R. & Miller, J. (1992) Risk and protective factors for alcohol and other drug problems in adolescence and early adulthood: implications for substance abuse prevention. *Psychological Bulletin, 112*, 64–105.

Hemmingssonm, T., Lundberg, I., Romelsjo, A. & Alfredsson, L. (1997) Alcoholism in social classes and occupations in Sweden. *International Journal of Epidemiology, 26*, 584–591.

Henry, B., Feehan, M., McGee, R., Stanton, W., Moffitt, T. & Silva, P. (1993) The importance of conduct problems and depressive symptoms in predicting adolescent substance use. *Journal of Abnormal Child Psychology, 21*, 469–480.

Henry, J.A. & Hill, I. (1998) Fatal interaction between ritonavir and MDMA. *Lancet, 352*, 1751–1752.

Hepatitis C Virus Projections Working Group (1998) *Estimates and projections of the hepatitis C virus epidemic in Australia.* Sydney: National Centre for HIV Epidemiology and Clinical Research, University of New South Wales.

Hickman, M., Madden, P., Henry, J., Baker, A., Wallace, C., Wakefield, J., Stimson, G. & Elliot, P. (2003) Trends in drug overdose deaths in England and Wales 1993–1998: methadone does not kill more people than heroin. *Addiction, 98*, 419–425.

Hidalgo, R.B. & Davidson, J.R.T. (2000) Posttraumatic stress disorder: epidemiology and health-related considerations. *Journal of Clinical Psychiatry, 61* (Suppl 7), 5–13.

Hien, D.A., Nunes, E., Levin, F.R. & Fraser, D. (2000) Posttraumatic stress disorder and short-term outcome in early methadone treatment. *Journal of Substance Abuse Treatment, 19*, 31–37.

Hindmarch I., Kerr, J.S. & Sherwood, N. (1991) The effects of alcohol and other drugs on psychomotor performance and cognitive function. *Alcohol and Alcoholism, 26*, 71–79.

Hoefler, M., Lieb, R., Perkonigg, A., Schuster, P., Sonntag, H. & Wittchen, H.U. (1999) Covariates of cannabis use progression in a representative population sample of adolescents: a prospective examination of vulnerability and risk factors. *Addiction, 94*, 1679–1694.

Hollander, J., Shih, R., Hoffman, R.S., Harchelroad, F.P., Phillips, S., Jeffrey, B., Kulig, K. & Thode, H.C. (1997) Predictors of artery disease in patients with cocaine-associated myocardial infarction. *American Journal of Medicine, 102*, 158–163.

Home Office (2004) *Tackling crack: a national plan.* London: Home Office.

Institute of Medicine (1996) *Pathways of addiction.* Washington: National Academy Press.

Hong, R., Matsuyama, E. & Nur, K. (1991) Cardiomyopathy associated with the smoking of crystal methamphetamine. *JAMA, 265*, 1152–1154.

Hopkins, D., Briss, P., Ricard, C., Husten, C., Carande-kulis, V. & Fielding, J. (2001) Reviews of evidence regarding interventions to reduce tobacco use and exposure to environmental tobacco smoke. *American Journal of Preventive Medicine, 20*, 16–66.

Hser, Y., Anglin, M.D. & Powers, K. (1993) A 24-year follow-up of California narcotic addicts. *Archives of General Psychiatry, 50*, 577–584.

Hser, Y., Grella, C., Chou, C.P. & Anglin, M.D. (1998) Relationship between drug treatment careers and outcomes: findings from the National Drug Abuse Treatment Outcome Study. *Evaluation Review, 22*, 496–519.

Hser, Y., Hoffman, V., Grella, C. & Anglin, M.D. (2001) A 33-year follow-up of narcotic addicts. *Archives of General Psychiatry, 58*, 503–508.

Huang, C.N., Wu, D.J. & Chen, K.S. (1993) Acute myocardial infarction caused by transnasal inhalation of amphetamine. *Japanese Heart Journal, 34*, 815–816.

Hubbard, R., Marsden, M., Rachal, J., Harwood, H., Cavanaugh, E. & Ginzburg, H. (1989) *Drug abuse treatment: A national study of effectiveness.* Chapel Hill, NC: University of North Carolina Press.

Hubbard R.L., Craddock, S.G., Flynn, P.M., Anderson, J. & Etheridge, R.M. (1997) Overview of one year follow-up outcomes in the Drug Abuse Treatment Outcome Study (DATOS). *Psychology of Addictive Behaviours, 11*, 261–278.

Hulse, G.K., English, D.R., Milne, E. & Holman, C.D.J. (1999) The quantification of mortality resulting from the regular use of illicit opiates. *Addiction, 94*, 221–229.

Hunt, N., Griffiths, P., Southwell, M., Stillwell, G. & Strang, J. (1999) Preventing and curtailing injecting drug use: a review of opportunities for developing and delivering "route transition interventions". *Drug and Alcohol Review, 18*, 441–445.

Hurley, S., Jolley, D.J. & Kaldor, J.M. (1997) Effectiveness of needle-exchange programmes for prevention of HIV infection. *Lancet, 349*, 1797–1800.

Jaffe, J.H. (1985) Drug addiction and drug abuse. In A. Goodman, T.W. Gilma, A.S. Nies & P. Taylor (Eds), *Goodman and Gilman's: the pharmacological basis of therapeutics (8th Edition)* (pp. 532–581). New York: McGrath Hill.

Jaffe, J.H. & Martin, W.R. (1985) Opioid analgesics and antagonists. In A.G. Gilman, T.W. Rall, A.S. Nies & P. Taylor (Eds), *The pharmacological basis of therapeutics* (8th Edition) (pp. 485–521). New York: Pergamon Press.

Jager, J., Limburg, W., Kretzschmar, M., Postma, M. & Wiessing, L. (Eds) (2004) *Hepatitis C and injecting drug use: Impact, costs and policy options. EMCDDA Monograph 7.* Luxembourg: Office for Official Publications of the European Communities.

Joe, G.W. & Simpson, D.D. (1987) Mortality rates among opioid addicts in a longitudinal study. *American Journal of Public Health, 77*, 347–348.

Joe, G.W., Lehman, W. & Simpson, D.D. (1982) Addict death rates during a four-year posttreatment follow-up. *American Journal of Public Health, 72*, 703–709.

Johnson, B. (2003) Patterns of drug distribution: implications and issues. *Substance Use & Misuse, 38*, 1789–1806.

Johnsson, E. & Fridell, M. (1997) Suicide attempts in a cohort of drug abusers: a five year follow-up study. *Acta Psychiatrica Scandinavia, 96*, 362–366.

Johnston, L.D., O'Malley, P. & Bachman, J.G. (2000a) National survey results on drug use from the monitoring the future study, 1975–1999. *College students and young adults ages 19–40* (Vol. 2) Rockville, MD: National Institute on Drug Abuse.

(2000b) National survey results on drug use from the monitoring the future study, 1975–1999. *Secondary school students* (Vol. 1) Rockville, MD: National Institute on Drug Abuse.

(2003) National survey results on drug use from the monitoring the future study, 1975–2003. Rockville, MD: National Institute on Drug Abuse.

Jones, A.W. & Holmgren, A. (2005) Abnormally high concentrations of amphetamine in blood of impaired drivers. *Journal of Forensic Sciences, 50*, 1215–1220.

Jones, C., Donnelly, N., Swift, W. & Weatherburn, D. (2005) *Driving under the influence of cannabis: the problem and potential countermeasures. Crime and Justice Bulletin No. 87.* Sydney: NSW Bureau of Crime Statistics and Research.

Jones, D.L., Irwin, K.L., Inciardi, J., Bowser, B., Schilling, R., Word, C., Evans, P., Faruque, S., McCoy, H. & Brian, R. (1998) The high-risk sexual practices of crack-moking sex workers recruited from the streets of three American Cities. *Sexually Transmitted Diseases, 25*, 187–193.

Jonnes, J. (1996) *Hep-Cats, Narcs and Pipe Dreams: A History of America's Romance with Illegal Drugs.* New York: Scribner.

Julien, R.M. (2001) *A Primer of Drug Action.* New York: Henry Holt and Company.

Kakko, J., Svanborg, D., Kreek, M.J. & Hellig, M. (2003) 1-year retention and social function after buprenorphine-assisted relapse prevention treatment for heroin dependence in Sweden: a randomised, placebo controlled trial. *Lancet, 361*, 662–668.

Kalant, H., Corrigall, W., Hall, W. & Smart, R. (Eds) (1999) *The Health Effects of Cannabis.* Toronto, Ont.: Centre for Addiction and Mental Health.

Kandel, D. (1991) The social demography of drug use. *Milbank Quarterly, 69*, 365–414.

Kandel, D., Chen, K., Warner, L.A., Kessler, R.C. & Grant, B. (1997) Prevalence and demographic correlates of symptoms of last year dependence on alcohol, nicotine, marijuana and cocaine in the US population. *Drug and Alcohol Dependence, 44*, 11–29.

Kandel, D.B., Yamaguchi, K. & Chen, K. (1992) Stages of progression in drug involvement from adolescence to adulthood: further evidence for the gateway theory. *Journal of Studies on Alcohol, 53*, 447–457.

Karch, S.B. (2002) *Karch's Pathology of Drug Abuse* (3rd Edition). Boca Raton, FL: CRC Press.

Karch, S.B., Stephens, M.D. & Ho, C.H. (1998) Relating cocaine blood concentrations to toxicity: an autopsy study of 99 cases. *Journal of Forensic Sciences, 43*, 41–45.

(1999) Methamphetamine–related deaths in San Francisco: demographic, pathologic and toxicologic findings. *Journal of Forensic Sciences, 44*, 359–368.

Kaye, S. & Darke, S. (2004) Non-fatal cocaine overdose among injecting and non-injecting cocaine users in Sydney, Australia. *Addiction, 99,* 1315–1322.

Kaye, S. & McKetin, R. (2005) *Cardiotoxicity associated with methamphetamine use and signs of cardiovascular pathology among methamphetamine users.* NDARC Technical Report No. 238. Sydney: National Drug and Alcohol Research Centre, University of New South Wales.

Kaye, S., Darke, S. & Finlay-Jones, R. (1998) The onset of heroin use and criminal behaviour: does order make a difference? *Drug and Alcohol Dependence*, *53*, 79–86.

Kelly, E., Darke, S. & Ross, J. (2004) A review of drug use and driving: epidemiology, impairment, risk factors and risk perceptions. *Drug and Alcohol Review*, *23*, 319–344.

Kendler, K.S. (1999) Preparing for gene discovery: a further agenda for psychiatry. *Archives of General Psychiatry*, *56*, 554–555.

Kendler, K., Neale, M., Sullivan, P., Corey, L., Gardner, C. & Prescott, C. (1999) A population-based twin study in women of smoking initiation and nicotine dependence. *Psychological Medicine*, *29*, 299–308.

Kendler, K.S. & Prescott, C.A. (1998a) Cannabis use, abuse, and dependence in a population-based sample of female twins. *American Journal of Psychiatry*, *155*, 1016–1022.

(1998b) Cocaine use, abuse and dependence in a population-based sample of female twins. *British Journal of Psychiatry*, *173*, 345–350.

Kerr, T., Palepu, A., Barnes, G., Walsh, J., Hogg, R., Montaner, J., Tyndall, M. & Wood, E. (2004) Psychosocial determinants of adherence to highly active antiretroviral therapy among injection drug users in Vancouver. *Antiviral Therapy*, *9*, 407–414.

Kerr, T., Small, W. & Wood, E. (2005) The public health and social impacts of drug market enforcement: a review of the evidence. *International Journal of Drug Policy*, *16*, 210–220.

Kessler, R.C., Sonnega, A., Bromet, E., Hughes, M. & Nelson, C.B. (1995) Posttraumatic stress disorder in the National Comorbidity Survey. *Archives of General Psychiatry*, *52*, 1048–1060.

Kiddorf, M., Brooner, R.K., King, V.L., Chutuape, M.A. & Stitzer, M.L. (1996) Concurrent validity of cocaine and sedative dependence diagnoses in opioid-dependent outpatients. *Drug and Alcohol Dependence*, *42*, 117–123.

Kimber, J., MacDonald, M., Van beek, I., Kaldor, J., Weatherburn, D., Lapsley, H. & Mattick, R.P. (2003) The Sydney medically supervised injecting centre: client characteristics and predictors of frequent attendance during the first 12 months of operation. *Journal of Drug Issues*, *33*, 639–648.

Kintz, P. (2001) Deaths involving buprenorphine: a compendium of French cases. *Forensic Science International*, *121*, 65–69.

Kintz, P., Mangin, P., Lugnier, A.A. & Chaumont, A.J. (1989) Toxicological data after heroin overdose. *Human Toxicology*, *8*, 487–489.

Kirchmayer, U., Davoli, M., Verster, A. D., Amato, L., Ferri, M. & Perucci, C. A. (2002) A systematic review on the efficacy of naltrexone maintenance treatment in opioid dependence. *Addiction*, *97*, 1241–1249.

Kjelsberg, E., Winther, M. & Dahl, A.A. (1995) Overdose deaths in young substance abusers: accidents or hidden suicides. *Acta Psychiatrica Scandinavia*, *91*, 236–242.

Klee, H. & Morris, J. (1995) Factors that characterize street injectors. *Addiction*, *90*, 837–841.

Klee, H., Faugier, J., Hayes, C., Boulton, T. & Morris, J. (1990) AIDS-related risk behaviour, polydrug use and temazepam. *British Journal of Addiction, 85,* 1125–1132.

Kontos, M.C., Jesse, R.L., Tatum, J.L. & Ornato, J.P. (2003) Coronary angiographic findings in patients with cocaine-associated chest pain. *Journal of Emergency Medicine, 24,* 9–13.

Kosten, T.R. & Rounsaville, B.J. (1988) Suicidality among opioid addicts: a 2.5 year follow-up. *American Journal of Drug and Alcohol Abuse, 14,* 357–369.

Kotler, P. & Zaltman, G. (1971) Social marketing: an approach to planned social change. *Journal of Marketing, 35,* 3–12.

Kreek, M.J. (1983) Factors modifying the pharmacological effectiveness of methadone. In J.R. Cooper, F. Altman, B.S. Brown & D. Czechowicz (Eds), *Research on the treatment of narcotic addiction: state of the art* (pp. 95–114). Rockville, MD: US Department of Health and Human Services.

Kreek, M.J. (1987) Tolerance and dependence: implications for the pharmacological treatment of addiction. In L.S. Harris (Ed.), *NIDA Research monograph 76 – problems of drug dependence 1986: proceeding of the 48th annual scientific meeting. The Committee on Problems of Drug Dependence, Inc.* (pp. 53–62). Rockville, MD: US Department of Health and Human Services.

Kronstrand, R., Grundin, R. & Jonsson, J. (1998) Incidence of opiates, amphetamines, and cocaine in hair and blood in fatal cases of heroin overdose. *Forensic Science International, 92,* 29–38.

Kuo, I. & Strathdee, S.A. (2005) After the flowers are gone … what happens next? *International Journal of Drug Policy, 16,* 112–114.

Laidler, K.A.J. & Morgan, P. (1997) Kinship and community: The "ice" crisis in Hawaii. In H. Klee (Ed.), *Amphetamine misuse:international perspectives on current trends* (pp. 163–179). Amsterdam: Harwood Academic Publishers.

Lan, K.C., Lin, Y.F., Yu, F.C., Lin, C.S. & Chu, P. (1998) Clinical manifestations and prognostic features of acute methamphetamine intoxication. *Journal of the Formosan Medical Association, 97,* 528–533.

Lange, R.A. & Hillis, L.D. (2001) Cardiovascular complications of cocaine use. *New England Journal of Medicine, 345,* 351–358.

Langendam, M.W., van Bussel, G.H.A., Coutinho, R.A. & van Ameijden, E.J.C. (2001) The impact of harm-reduction-based methadone treatment on mortality among heroin users. *American Journal of Public Health, 91,* 774–780.

Lauer, G.M. & Walker, B. (2001) Hepatitis C infection. *New England Journal of Medicine, 345,* 41–52.

Law, M., Dore, G., Bath, N., Thompson, S., Crofts, N., Dolan, K., Giles, W., Gow, P., Kaldor, J., Loveday, S., Powell, E., Spencer, J. & Wodak, A. (2003) Modelling hepatitis C virus incidence, prevalence and long-term sequelae in Australia, 2001. *International Journal of Epidemiology, 32,* 717–724.

Leimer, N., Hofmann, P. & Chaudrey, H.R. (1994) Nasal administration of naloxone is as effective as the intravenous route in opiate addicts. *International Journal of the Addictions, 29*, 819–827.

Lenton, S.R. & Hargreaves, K.M. (2000a) Should we conduct a trial of distributing naloxone to heroin users for peer administration to prevent fatal overdose? *Medical Journal of Australia, 173*, 260–263.

(2000b) A trial of naloxone to heroin users for peer administration has merit, but will the lawyers let it happen? *Drug and Alcohol Review, 9*, 365–369.

Limburg, W. (2004) Natural history, treatment and prevention of hepatitis C in injecting drug users: an overview. In J. Jager, W. Limburg, M. Kretzschmar, M. Postma & L. Wiessing (Eds), *Hepatitis C and injecting drug use: Impact, costs and policy options. EMCDDA Monograph 7* (pp. 21–38). Luxembourg: Office for Official Publications of the European Communities.

Ling, W., Wesson, D.R., Charuvastra, C. & Klett, C.J. (1996) A controlled trial comparing buprenorphine and methadone maintenance in opioid dependence. *Archives of General Psychiatry, 53*, 401–407.

Loeber, R., Southamer-Lober, M. & White, H. (1999) Developmental aspects of delinquency and internalising problems and their association with persistent juvenile substance use between ages 7 and 18. *Journal of Clinical Child Psychology, 28*, 322–332.

Logan, B.K., Fligner, C.L. & Haddix, T. (1998) Cause and manner of death in fatalities involving methamphetamine. *Journal of Forensic Sciences, 43*, 28–34.

Longo, M., Hunter, C., Lokan, R., White, J. & White, M. (2000) The prevalence of alcohol, cannabinoids, benzodiazepines and stimulants amongst injured drivers and their role in driver culpability. Part 2: the relationship between drug prevalence and drug concentration, and driver culpability. *Accident Analysis and Prevention, 32*, 623–632.

Lora-Tamayo, C., Tena, T. & Rodriguez, A. (1997) Amphetamine derivative related deaths. *Forensic Science International, 85*, 149–157.

Loxley, W. (1998) Weed or speed? Convicted drug dealers' views of substitutions in the Western Australian illicit drug market to 1992. *International Journal of Drug Policy, 9*, 109–118.

Lucas, G.M., Cheever, L.W., Chaisson, R.E. & Moore, R.D. (2001) Detrimental effects of continued illicit drug use on the treatment of HIV-1 infection. *Journal of Acquired Immune Deficiency Syndromes: Journal of Acquired Immune Deficiency Syndromes, 27*, 251–259.

Lucas, G.M., Gebo, K.A., Chaisson, R.E. & Moore, R.D. (2002) Longitudinal assessment of the effects of drug and alcohol abuse on HIV-1 treatment outcomes in an urban clinic. *AIDS, 16*, 767–774.

Lucas, J., Goldfeder, L.B. & Gill, J.R. (2002) Bodies found in the waterways of New York City. *Journal of Forensic Science, 47*, 137–141.

Luthar, S.S., Cushing, G. & Rounsaville, B.J. (1996) Gender differences among opioid abusers: pathways to disorder and profiles of psychopathology. *Drug and Alcohol Dependence, 43, 179–189.*

Lyles, C., Graham, N.M., Astemborski, J., Vlahov, D., Margolick, J., Saah, A. & Farzadegan, H. (1999) Cell-associated infectious HIV-1 viral load as a predictor of clinical progression and survival among HIV-1 infected injection drug users and homosexual men. *European Journal of Epidemiology, 15,* 99–108.

Lynskey, M. & Hall, W. (2000a) The effects of adolescent cannabis use on educational attainment: a review. *Addiction, 95,* 1621–1630.

Lynskey, M., Degenhardt, L. & Hall, W. (2000b) Cohort trends in youth suicide in Australia. *Australian and New Zealand Journal of Psychiatry, 34,* 408–412.

Lynskey, M., Glowinski, A.L., Todoraov, A., Bucholz, K.K., Madden, P.A.F., Nelson, E.C., Statham, D.J., Martin, N.G. & Heath, A.C. (2004) Major depressive disorder, suicidal ideation, and suicide attempts in twins discordant for cannabis dependence and early-onset cannabis use. *Archives of General Psychiatry, 61,* 1026–1032.

Lynskey, M.T., Fergusson, D. & Horwood, L.J. (1998) The origins of the correlations between tobacco, alcohol, and cannabis use during adolescence. *Journal of Child Psychology and Psychiatry, 39,* 995–1005.

MacLean, S. & D'Abbs, P. (2002) Petrol sniffing in Aboriginal communities: a review of interventions. *Drug and Alcohol Review, 21,* 65–71.

Madianos, M.G., Gefou-Madianou, D. & Stefanis, C.N. (1994) Symptoms of depression, suicidal behaviours and use of substances in Greece: a nationwide general population survey. *Acta Psychiatrica Scandinavia, 89,* 159–166.

Maher, L. (2002) Don't leave me this way: ethnography and injecting drug use in the age of AIDS. *International Journal of Drug Policy, 13,* 311–325.

Maher, L. & Dixon, D. (1999) Policing and public health: law enforcement and harm minimization in a street-level drug market. *British Journal of Criminology, 39,* 488–512. (2001) The cost of crackdowns: policing cabramatta's heroin market. *Current Issues in Criminal Justice, 13,* 5–22.

Maher, L., Swift, W. & Dawson, M. (2001) Heroin purity and composition in Sydney, Australia. *Drug and Alcohol Review, 20,* 439–448.

Maier, I. & Wu, G.Y. (2002) Hepatitis C and HIV co-infection: a review. *World Journal of Gastroenterology, 8,* 577–579.

Makkai, T. & McAllister, I. (1998) *Patterns of drug use in Australia, 1985–1995.* Canberra: Australian Government Publishing Service.

Man, L.H., Berst, D., Gossop, M., Noble, A. & Strang, J. (2002) Risk of overdose: do those who witness most overdoses also experience most overdoses? *Journal of Substance Use, 7,* 136–140.

Manning, F.J., Ingraham, L.H., Derouin, E.M., Vaughn, M.S., Kukura, F.C. & St Michel, G.R. (1983) Drug "overdoses" among US soldiers in Europe, 1978–1979. II. Psychological autopsies following deaths and near-deaths, *International Journal of the Addictions, 18,* 153–156.

Manns, M.P., McHutchinson, J., Gordon, S., Schiff, E. R., Shiffman, M., Lee, W., Rustgi, V., Goodman, Z.D., Ling, M., Cort, S. & Albrecht, J. (2001) PEG interferon alfa-2b in combination with ribavirin compared to interferon alfa-2b plus ribavirin for initial treatment for chronic hepatitis C. *Lancet*, *358*, 958–965.

Manski, C., Pepper, J.V. & Petrie, C.V. (2001) *Informing America's policy on illegal drugs: what we don't know keeps hurting us*. Washington DC: National Academy Press.

Marmor, M., Des Jarlais, D.C., Cohen, H., Friedman, S.R., Beatrice, S.T., Dubin, N., El-Sadr, W., Mildvan, D., Yankovitz, S., Mathur, V. & Holzman, R. (1987) Risk factors for infection of human immunodeficiency virus among intravenous drug abusers in New York City. *AIDS*, *1*, 39–44.

Martyres, R.F., Clode, D. & Burns, J.M. (2004) Seeking drugs or seeking help? Escalating "doctor shopping" by young heroin users before fatal overdose. *Medical Journal of Australia*, *180*, 211–214.

Marx, A., Schick, M.T. & Minder, C.E. (1994) Drug-related mortality in Switzerland from 1987 to 1989 in comparison to other countries. *International Journal of the Addictions*, *29*, 837–860.

Marzuk, P., Tardiff, K., Leon, A., Stajic, M., Morgan, E. & Mann, J. (1990) Prevalence of recent cocaine use among motor vehicle fatalities in New York City. *JAMA*, *263*, 250–256.

Marzuk, P., Tardiff, K., Leon, A., Hirsch, C.S., Stajic, M., Portera, L. & Hartwell, N. (1997) Poverty and fatal accidental drug overdoses of cocaine and opiates in New York City: an ecological study. *American Journal of Drug and Alcohol Abuse*, *23*, 221–228.

Marzuk, P.M., Tardiff, K., Leon, A., Hirsch, C.S., Stajic, M., Portera, L., Hartwell, N. & Iqbal, M.I. (1995) Fatal injuries after cocaine use as a leading cause of death among young adults in New York City. *New England Journal of Medicine*, *332*, 1753–1757.

Massing, M. (2000) *The Fix*. Berkeley, CA: University of California Press.

Matsumoto, T., Kanai, T. & Takeuchi, N. (2000) Clinical features of adolescent methamphetamine abusers: current pattern of methamphetamine use, *Japanese Journal of Child and Adolescent Psychiatry*, *41*, 19–31.

Mattick, R., Digiusto, E., Doran, C., O'Brien, S., Shanahan, M., Kimber, J., Henderson, N., Breen, C., Shearer, J., Gates, J., Shakeshaft, A. & NEPOD trial investigators (2001) *national evaluation of pharmacotherapies for opioid dependence (NEPOD): report of results and recommendations*. Sydney: National Drug and Alcohol Research Centre, University of New South Wales.

Mattick, R.P., Ali, R., White, J., O'Brien, S., Wolk, S. & Danz, C. (2003) Buprenorphine versus methadone maintenance therapy: a randomized double-blind trial with 405 opioid-dependent patients. *Addiction*, *98*, 441–452.

Mattick, R.P., Breen, C., Kimber, J. & Davoli, M. (2003a) Methadone maintenance therapy versus no opioid replacement therapy for opioid dependence. *The Cochrane Database of Systematic Reviews*.

Mattick, R.P., Kimber, J., Breen, C. & Davoli, M. (2003b) Buprenorphine maintenance versus placebo or methadone maintenance for opioid dependence. *The Cochrane Database of Systematic Reviews*.

Maxwell, J.C., Pullum, T.W. & Tannert, K. (2005) Deaths of clients in methadone treatment in Texas, 1994–2002. *Drug and Alcohol Dependence, 78*, 73–81.

May, T. & Hough, M. (2001) Illegal dealings: the impact of low-level police enforcement on drug markets. *European Journal on Criminal Policy and Research, 9*, 137–162.

McAnulty, J.M., Tesselaar, H. & Fleming, D.W. (1995) Mortality among injection drug users identified as "out of treatment". *American Journal of Public Health, 85*, 119–120.

McBride, N. (2003) A systematic review of school drug education. *Health Education Research Theory and Practice, 18*, 729–742.

McCance-Katz, E.F., Jatlow, P., Rainey, P. & Friedland, G. (1998) Methadone effects on zidovudine (AZT) disposition (ACTG 262) *Journal of Acquired Immune Deficiency Syndrome and Human Retrovirology, 18*, 435–443.

McCance-Katz, E.F., Gourevitch, M.N., Arnsten, J., Sarlo, J., Rainey, P. & Jatlow, P. (2002) Modified directly observed therapy (MDOT) for injection drug users with HIV disease. *American Journal of the Addictions, 11*, 271–278.

McGregor, C., Darke, S., Christie, P. & Ali, R. (1998) Experience of non-fatal overdose among heroin users in Adelaide: circumstances and risk perception. *Addiction, 93*, 701–711.

McGregor, C., Ali, R., Christie, P. & Darke, S. (2001) Overdose among heroin users: evaluation of an intervention in South Australia. *Addiction Research, 9*, 481–501.

McGregor, C., Ali, R., Lokan, R., Christie, P. & Darke, S. (2002) Accidental fatalities among heroin users in South Australia, 1994–1997: toxicological findings and circumstances of death. *Addiction Research and Theory, 10*, 335–346.

McHutchinson, J., Gordon, S., Schiff, E.R., Shiffman, M., Lee, W., Rustgi, V., Goodman, Z.D., Ling, M., Cort, S. & Albrecht, J. (1998) Interferon alfa-2b alone or in combination with ribavirin as initial treatment for chronic hepatitis C. Hepatitis Interventional Therapy Group. *New England Journal of Medicine, 339*, 1485–1492.

McKetin, R., McLaren, J. & Kelly, E. (2005a) *The Sydney methamphetamine market: patterns of supply, use, personal harms and social consequences. National drug law enforcement research fund monograph no. 13.* Adelaide: Australasian Centre for Policing Studies.

McKetin, R., McLaren, J., Kelly, E., Hall, W. & Hickman, M. (2005b) *Estimating the number of regular and dependent methamphetamine users in Australia. NDARC Technical Report No. 172.* Sydney: National Drug and Alcohol Research Centre, University of New South Wales.

Medrano, M.A., Zule, W.A., Hatch, J. & Desmond, D.P. (1999) Prevalence of childhood trauma in a community sample of substance-abusing women. *American Journal of Drug and Alcohol Abuse, 25*, 449–462.

Mendelson, J., Jones, R.T., Upton, R. & Jacob, P. (1995) Methamphetamine and ethanol interactions in humans. *Clinical Pharmacology and Therapeutics, 57*, 559–568.

Mesquita, F., Kral, A., Reingold, A., Haddad, I., Sanches, M., Turienzo, G., Piconez, D., Araujo, P. & Bueno, R. (2001) Overdoses among cocaine users in Brazil. *Addiction*, *96*, 1809–1813.

Metzger, D.S., Woody, G.E., McLellan, A.T., O'Brien, C.P., Druley, P., Navaline, H., DePhillipis, D., Stolly, P. & Abrutyn, E. (1993) Human immunodeficiency virus seroconversion among intravenous drug users in- and out-of-treatment: an 18-month prospective follow-up. *Journal of Acquired Immune Deficiency Syndromes*, *6*, 1049–1055.

Metzger, D.S., Navaline, H. & Woody, G.E. (1998) Drug abuse treatment as AIDS prevention. *Public Health Reports*, *113* (Suppl 1), 97–106.

(2000) The role of drug abuse treatment in the prevention of HIV infection. In J.L. Peterson & R.J. DiClemente (Eds), *Handbook of HIV prevention AIDS prevention and mental health* (pp. 147–157). Netherlands: Kluwer Academic Publishers.

Miech, R., Chilcoat, H. & Harder, V. (2005) The increase in the association of education and cocaine use over the 1980s and 1990s: evidence for a "historical period" effect. *Drug and Alcohol Dependence*, *79*, 311–320.

Milby, J.B., Sims, M.K., Khuder, S., Schumachere, J.E. & Huggins, N. (1996) Psychiatric comorbidity; prevalence in methadone maintenance treatment. *American Journal of Drug and Alcohol Abuse*, *22*, 95–107.

Miles, C.P. (1977) Conditions predisposing to suicide: a review. *Journal of Nervous and Mental Disease*, *164*, 231–246.

Mills, K., Lynskey, M., Teesson, M., Ross, J. & Darke, S. (2005) Post-traumatic stress disorder among people with heroin dependence in the Australian Treatment Outcome Study (ATOS): prevalence and correlates. *Drug and Alcohol Dependence*, *77*, 243–249.

Mills, K.L., Teesson, M., Darke, S., Ross, J. & Lynskey, M. (2004) Young people with heroin dependence: Findings from the Australian Treatment Outcome Study (ATOS). *Journal of Substance Abuse Treatment*, *27*, 67–73.

Minozzi, S., Amato, L., Vecchi, S., Davoli, M., Kirchmayer, U. & Verster, A. (2006) Naltrexone maintenance treatment for opioid dependence. *The Cochrane Database of Systematic Reviews*.

Mintzer, M.Z. & Griffiths, R.R. (1999) Triazolam and zolpidem: effects on human memory and attentional processes. *Psychopharmacology*, *144*, 8–19.

Miotto, K., McCann, M.J., Rawson, R.A., Frosch, D. & Ling, W. (1997) Overdose, suicide attempts and death among a cohort of naltrexone-treated opioid addicts. *Drug and Alcohol Dependence*, *45*, 131–134.

Mittleman, M.A, Mintzer, D., Maclure, M., Tofler, G.H., Sherwood, J. & Muller, J. (1999) Triggering of myocardial infarction by cocaine. *Circulation*, *99*, 2737–2741.

Mittleman, M.A., Lewis, R.A., Maclure, M., Sherwood, J.B. & Muller, J.E. (2001) Triggering myocardial infarction by marijuana. *Circulation*, *103*, 2805–2809.

Moliterno, D.J., Willard, J.E., Negus, B.H., Boehrer, J.D., Glamann, D.B., Landau, C., Rossen, J., Winniford, M.D. & Hillis, L.D. (1994) Coronary-artery vasoconstriction induced by cocaine, cigarette smoking or both. *New England Journal of Medicine*, *330*, 454–459.

Monforte, J.R. (1977) Some observations concerning blood morphine concentrations in narcotic addicts. *Journal of Forensic Sciences*, *22*, 718–724.

Montoya, I.D., Umbricht, A. & Preston, K.L. (1995) Buprenorphine for human immunovirus-positive opiate-dependent patients. *Biological Psychiatry*, *38*, 135–136.

Morgan, P. & Beck, J. (1997) The legacy and the paradox: hidden contexts of methamphetamine use in the United States. In H. Klee (Ed.), *Amphetamine misuse: international perspectives on current trends* (pp. 135–162). The Netherlands: Harwood Academic Publishers.

Muntaner, C., Eaton, W.W., Dialai, C., Kessler, R.C. & Sorlie, P.D. (1998) Social class, assets, organizational control and the prevalence of common groups of psychiatric disorders. *Social Science and Medicine*, *47*, 2043–2053.

Murphy, E., Collier, A. & Kalish, L. (2002) Highly active antiretroviral therapy decreases mortality and morbidity in patients with advanced HIV disease. *Annals of Internal Medicine*, *135*, 17–26.

Murphy, S.L., Rounsaville, B.J., Eyre, S. & Kleber, H.D. (1983) Suicide attempts in treated opiate addicts. *Comprehensive Psychiatry*, *24*, 79–89.

Musto, D.F. & Ramos, M.R. (1981) A follow-up study of the New Haven morphine maintenance clinic of 1920. *New England Journal of Medicine*, *304*, 1071–1077.

National Centre in HIV Epidemiology and Clinical Research (2003) *HIV/AIDS, viral hepatitis and sexually transmissible infections in Australia Annual Surveillance Report 2002.* Sydney, NSW: National Centre in HIV Epidemiology and Clinical Research, University of New South Wales.

National Drug Intelligence Centre (2003) *National drug threat assessment 2003.* Johnstown, PA: US Department of Justice, National Drug Intelligence Centre.

National Institute on Drug Abuse (2003) *Epidemiologic trends in drug abuse.* Community Epidemiology Work Group. Rockville, MD: Department of Health and Human Services.

National Research Council and Institute of Medicine (2000) *From neurons to neighbourhoods: The science of early childhood development.* Washington, DC: National Academy Press.

Neaigus, A., Miller, M., Friedman, S., Hagen, D.L., Sifaneck, S.J., Ildefonso, G. & Des Jarlais, D.C. (2001) Potential risk factors for the transition to injecting among non-injecting heroin users: a comparison of former injectors and never injectors. Addiction, *96*, 847–860.

Neale, J. (2000) Suicidal intent in non-fatal illicit drug overdose. *Addiction*, *95*, 85–93.

Neale, J. & Robertson, M. (2005) Recent life problems and non-fatal overdose among heroin users entering treatment. *Addiction*, *100*, 168–175.

Newcomb, M.D., Maddahian, E. & Bentler, P.M. (1986) Risk factors for drug use among adolescents: concurrent and longitudinal analyses. *American Journal of Public Health*, *76*, 525–531.

Norris, F.H. (1992) Epidemiology of trauma: frequency and impact of different potentially traumatic events on different demographic groups. *Journal of Consulting and Clinical Psychology*, *60*, 409–418.

Norstrom, T. & Skog, O.J. (2003) Saturday opening of alcohol retail shops in Sweden: an impact analysis. *Journal of Studies on Alcohol*, *64*, 393–401.

Novick, D.M., Joseph, H., Croxson, T.S., Salsitz, E.A., Wang, G., Richman, B.L., Porestski, L., Keefe, J.B. & Whimbey, E. (1990) Absence of antibody to human immunodeficiency virus in long-term, socially rehabilitated methadone maintenance patients. *Archives of Internal Medicine*, *150*, 97–99.

Obadia, Y., Perrin, V., Feroni, I., Vlahov, D. & Moatti, J. (2001) Injecting misuse of buprenorphine among French drug users. *Addiction*, *96*, 267–272.

Ochoa, K.C., Hahn, J.A., Seal, K.H. & Moss, A.R. (2001) Overdosing among young injection drug users in San Francisco. *Addictive Behaviors*, *26*, 453–460.

O'Doherty, M. & Farrington, A. (1997) Estimating local opioid addict mortality. *Addiction Research*, *4*, 321–327.

Office of National Statistics (2004) *Mortality statistics: general. Review of the registrar general on deaths in England and Wales, 2002*. London: Office of National Statistics.

Ogilvie, D., Gruer, L. & Haw, S. (2005) Young people's access to tobacco, alcohol, and other drugs. *British Medical Journal*, *331*, 393–396.

O'Kane, C.J., Tutt, D.C. & Bauer, L.A. (2002) Cannabis and driving: a new perspective. *Emergency Medicine*, *14*, 296–303.

Oliver, P., Horspool, M. & Keen, J. (2005) Fatal opiate overdose following regimen changes in naltrexone treatment. *Addiction*, *100*, 560–561.

Om, A., Elahham, S., Vestrovec, G.W., Guard, C., Reese, S. & Nixon, J.V. (1993) Left ventricular hypertrophy in normotensive cocaine users. *American Heart Journal*, *125*, 1441–1443.

O'Neill, W.M., Hanks, G.W., Simpson, P., Fallon, M.T., Jenkins, E. & Wesnes, K. (2000) The cognitive and psychomotor effects of morphine in healthy subjects:a randomised controlled trial of repeated (four) oral doses of dextropropoxyphene, morphine, lorazepam and placebo. *Pain*, *85*, 209–215.

Oppenheimer, E., Tobutt, C., Taylor, C. & Andrew, T. (1994) Death and survival in a cohort of heroin addicts from London clinics: a 22 year follow-up. *Addiction*, *89*, 1299–1308.

Orti, R.M., Domingo-Salvany, A., Munoz, A., MacFarlane, D., Suelves, J.M. & Anto, J.M. (1996) Mortality trends in a cohort of opiate addicts, Catalona, Spain. *International Journal of Epidemiology*, *25*, 545–553.

Orzel, J.A. (1982) Acute myocardial infarction complicated by chronic amphetamine use. *Archives of Internal Medicine*, *142*, 644.

Oyefesso, A., Ghodse, H., Clancy, C. & Corkery, J.M. (1999a) Suicide among drug addicts in the UK. *British Journal of Psychiatry*, *175*, 277–282.

Oyefesso, A., Ghodse, H., Clancy, C., Corkery, J.M. & Goldfinch, R. (1999b) Drug-related mortality: a study of teenage addicts over a 20-year period. *Social Psychiatry and Psychiatric Epidemiology*, *34*, 437–441.

Pachar, J.V. & Cameron, J.M. (1992) Submersion cases: a retrospective study. *Medicine Science and the Law*, *32*, 15–17.

Patton, G., Bond, L., Butler, H. & Glover, S. (2003) Changing schools, changing health? Design and implementation of the Gatehouse project. *Journal of Adolescent Health*, *33*, 231–239.

Perez-Jimenez, J.P. & Robert, M.S. (1997) Transitions in the route of heroin use. *European Addiction Research*, *3*, 93–98.

Perez-Reyes, M., Reid White, W., McDonald, S.A., Hicks, R.E., Jeffcoat, A.R., Hill, J.M. & Cook, C.E. (1991) Clinical effects of daily methamphetamine administration. *Clinical Neuropharmacology*, *14*, 352–358.

Perret, G., Deglon, J., Kreek, M.J., Ho, A. & La Harpe, R. (2000) Lethal methadone intoxications in Geneva, Switzerland, from 1994–1998. *Addiction*, *95*, 1647–1653.

Persaud, N.E., Klaskala, W., Tewari, T., Shultz, J. & Baum, M. (1999) Drug use and syphilis – Co-factors for HIV transmission among commercial sex workers in Guyana. *West Indian Medical Journal*, *48*, 52–56.

Perucci, C.A., Davoli, M., Rapiti, E., Abeni, D.D. & Forastieri, F. (1991) Mortality of intravenous drug users in Rome: a cohort study. *American Journal of Public Health*, *81*, 1307–1310.

Petronis, K.R. & Anthony, J.C. (2003) A different kind of contextual effect: geographical clustering of cocaine incidence in the USA. *Journal of Epidemiology and Community Health*, *57*, 893–900.

Petronis, K.R., Samuels, J.F., Moscicki, E.K. & Anthony, J.C. (1990) An epidemiologic investigation of potential risk factors for suicide attempts. *Social Psychiatry and Psychiatric Epidemiology*, *25*, 193–199.

Pettiti, D.B., Sidney, S., Quesenberry, C. & Bernstein, A. (1998) Stroke and cocaine or amphetamine use. *Epidemiology*, *9*, 596–600.

Pirkis, J., Burgess, P. & Dunt, D. (2000) Suicidal ideation and suicide attempts among Australian adults. *Crisis*, *21*, 16–25.

Pirnay, S., Borron, S.W., Guidecelli, C.P., Tourneau, J., Baud, F.J. & Ricordel, I. (2004) A critical review of the causes of death among post-mortem toxicological investigations: analysis of 34 buprenorphine-associated and 35 methadone-associated deaths. *Addiction*, *99*, 978–988.

Platt, J.J. (1997) *Cocaine Addiction. Theory, Research and Treatment*. Cambridge, MA: Harvard University Press.

Pokorny, A.D. (1983) Prediction of suicide in psychiatric patients. *Archives of General Psychiatry*, *40*, 249–257.

Polettini, A., Poloni, V., Groppi, A., Stramesi, C. Vignali, C., Politi, L. & Montagna, M. (2005) The role of cocaine in heroin-related deaths. Hypothesis on the interaction between heroin and cocaine. *Forensic Science International*, *153*, 23–28.

Pollack, H. & Heimer, R. (2004) The impact and cost-effectiveness of methadone maintenance treatment in preventing HIV and hepatitis C. In J. Jager, W. Limburg, M. Kretzschmar, M. Postma & L. Wiessing (Eds), *Hepatitis C and injecting drug use: impact, costs and policy options. EMCDDA Monograph 7* (pp. 345–370). Luxembourg: Office for Official Publications of the European Communities.

Pottieger, A.E., Tressell, P.A., Inciardi, J.A. & Rosales, T.A. (1992) Cocaine use patterns and overdose. *Journal of Psychoactive Drugs, 24*, 399–410.

Poulton, R., Caspi, A., Milne, B.J., Thomson, W.M., Taylor, A., Sears, M.R. & Moffitt, T.E. (2002) Association between children's experience of socioeconomic disadvantage and adult health: a life-course study. *Lancet, 360*, 1640–1645.

Powis, B., Strang, J., Griffiths, P., Taylor, C., Williamson, S., Fountain, J. & Gossop, M. (1999) Self-reported overdose among injecting drug users in London: extent and nature of the problem. Addiction, *94*, 471–478.

Poynard, T. (2004) Recent developments in hepatitis C diagnostics and treatment. In J. Jager, W. Limburg, M. Kretzschmar, M. Postma & L. Wiessing (Eds), *Hepatitis C and injecting drug use: impact, costs and policy options. EMCDDA Monograph 7* (pp. 41–76). Luxembourg: Office for Official Publications of the European Communities.

Preti, A., Miotto, P. & DeCoppi, M. (2002) Deaths by unintentional illicit drug overdose in Italy, 1984–2000. *Drug and Alcohol Dependence, 66*, 275–282.

Pritzker, D., Kanungo, A., Kilicarslan, T., Tyndale, R. & Sellers, E. (2002) Designer drugs that are potent inhibitors of CYP2D6. *Journal of Clinical Psychopharmacology, 22*, 330–332.

Quaglio, G., Talamini, G., Lechi, A., Venturini, L., Lugoboni, F., Gruppo Intersert Di Collaborazione Scientifica & Mezzelani, P. (2001) Study of heroin-related deaths in north-eastern Italy 1985–98 to establish main causes of death. *Addiction, 96*, 127–137.

Ragland, A.S., Ismail, Y. & Arsura, E.L. (1993) Myocardial infarction after amphetamine use. *American Heart Journal, 125*, 247–249.

Raikos, N., Tsoukali, H., Psaroulis, D., Vassiliadis, N., Tsoungas, M. & Njau, S.N. (2002) Amphetamine derivative related deaths in northern Greece. *Forensic Science International, 128*, 31–34.

Ravndal, E. & Vaglum, P. (1999) Overdoses and suicide attempts: different relations to psychopathology and substance abuse? A 5-year prospective study of drug abusers. *European Addiction Research, 5*, 63–70.

Reback, C.J., Larkins, S. & Shoptaw, S. (2003) Methamphetamine abuse as a barrier to HIV medication adherence among gay and bisexual men. *AIDS Care, 15*, 775–785.

Rehm, J., Room, R., Montiero, M., Gmel, G., Graham, K., Rehn, N., Sempos, C., Frick, U. & Jernigan, D. (2004) Alcohol use. Comparative quantification of health risks. In M. Ezzati, A. Lopez, A. Rodgers & C.J.L. Murray (Eds), *Comparative quantification of health risks. Global and regional burden of disease attributable to selected major risk factors*, Vol. 1 (pp 959–1108). Geneva: World Health Organization.

Rehm, J., Frick, U., Hartwig, C., Gutzwiller, F., Gschwend, P. & Uchtenhagen, A. (2005) Mortality in heroin-assisted treatment in Switzerland 1994–2000. *Drug and Alcohol Dependence, 79*, 137–143.

Reid, G. & Costigan, G. (2002) *Revisiting "The Hidden Epidemic": A situation assessment of drug use in Asia in the context of HIV/AIDS*. Melbourne: The MacFarlane Burnet Institute for Medical Research and Public Health.

Reynaud, M., Petti, G., Potard, D. & Courty, P. (1998) Six deaths linked to concomitant use of buprenorphine and benzodiazepines. *Addiction, 93*, 1385–1392.

Rhodes, T. & Simic, M. (2005) Transition and the HIV risk environment. *British Medical Journal, 331*, 220–223.

Rich, C.L., Ricketts, J.E., Fowler, R.C. & Young, D. (1988) Some differences between men and women who commit suicide. *American Journal of Psychiatry, 145*, 718–722.

Richards, J.R., Bretz, S.W., Johnson, E.B., Turnipseed, S.D., Brofeldt, B.T. & Derlet, R.W. (1999) Methamphetamine abuse and emergency department utilization. *The Western Journal of Medicine, 170*, 198–202.

Risser, D., Uhl, A., Stichenwirth, M., Honigschnabl, S., Hirz, W., Schneider, B., Stellwag-Carion, C., Klupp, N., Vycudilik, W. & Bauer, G. (2000) Quality of heroin and heroin-related deaths from 1987 to 1995 in Vienna, Austria. *Addiction, 95*, 375–382.

Robbe, H.W.J. & O'Hanlon, J.F. (1999) Marijuana, alcohol and actual driving performance. Washington: US Department of Transportation, National Traffic Safety Administration.

Rogers, C. (1993) Gang-related homicides in Los Angeles County. *Journal of Forensic Science, 38*, 831–834.

Robertson, J.R., Ronald, P.J.M., Raab, G., Ross, A.J. & Parpia, T. (1994) Deaths, HIV infection, abstinence, and other outcomes in a cohort of injecting drug users followed up for 10 years. *British medical Journal, 309*, 369–372.

Robins, L. (1978) Sturdy childhood predictors of adult anti-social behavior: replications from longitudinal studies. *Psychological Medicine, 8*, 611–622.

Room, R., Babor, T. & Rehm, J. (2005) Alcohol and public health. *Lancet, 365*, 519–530.

Ross, J. & Darke, S. (2000) The nature of benzodiazepine dependence among heroin users in Sydney, Australia. *Addiction, 95*, 1785–1793.

Ross, J., Darke, S. & Hall, W. (1996) Benzodiazepine use among heroin users in Sydney: patterns, availability and procurement. *Drug and Alcohol Review, 15*, 237–243.

Ross, M., Wodak, A., Loxley, W., Stowe, A. & Drury, M. (1992) *Staying negative. Summary of the results of the Australian National AIDS and Injecting Drug Use Study*. Sydney: University of New South Wales.

Rossow, I. (1994) Suicide among drug addicts in Norway. *Addiction, 89*, 1667–1673.

Rossow, I. & Lauritzen, G. (1999) Balancing on the edge of death: suicide attempts and life-threatening overdoses among drug addicts. *Addiction, 94*, 209–219.

(2001) Shattered childhood: a key issue in suicidal behavior among drug addicts. *Addiction, 96*, 227–240.

Roxburgh, A., Degenhardt, L. & Breen, C. (2004) Changes in patterns of drug use among injecting drug users following a reduction in the availability of heroin in New South Wales, Australia. *Drug and Alcohol Review, 23*, 287–294.

Roy, A. (2001) Characteristics of cocaine-dependent patients who attempt suicide. *American Journal of Psychiatry*, *158*, 1215–1219.

    (2002) Characteristics of opiate dependent patients who attempt suicide. *Journal of Clinical Psychiatry*, *63*, 403–407.

Rubin, V. & Comitas, L. (1975) *Ganja in Jamaica: medical anthropological study of chronic marihuana se*. The Hague: Mouton.

Ruttenber, A.J. & Luke, J.L. (1984) Heroin-related deaths: new epidemiologic insights. *Science*, *226*, 14–20.

Ruttenber, A.J, Kalter, H.O. & Santinga, P. (1990) The role of ethanol abuse in the etiology of heroin-related death. *Journal of Forensic Sciences*, *35*, 891–900.

Sanchez, J., Rodriguez, B., Fuente, L., Barrio, G., Vicente, J., Roca, J. & Royuela, L. (1995) Opiates or cocaine: mortality from acute reactions in six major Spanish cities. *Journal of Epidemiology and Community Health*, *49*, 54–60.

Sanchez-Carbonell, X. & Seus, L. (2000) Ten-year survival analysis of a cohort of heroin addicts in Catalonia: the EMETYST project. *Addiction*, *95*, 941–948.

Schifano, F. (2004) A bitter pill. Overview of ecstasy (MDMA, MDA) related fatalities. *Psychopharmacology*, *173*, 242–248.

Schifano, F., Oyefesso, A., Corkery, J., Cobain, K., Jambert-Gray, R., Martinotti, G. & Ghodse, A.H. (2003a) Death rates from ecstasy (MDMA, MDA) and polydrug use in England and Wales, 1996–2002. *Psychopharmacology*, *18*, 519–524.

Schifano, F., Oyefesso, A., Webb, L., Pollard, M., Corkery, J. & Ghodse, A.H. (2003b) Review of deaths related to taking ecstasy, England and Wales, 1997–2000. *British Medical Journal*, *326*, 80–81.

Schoenbaum, E.E., Hartel, D., Selwyn, P.A., Klein, R.S., Davenny, K., Rogers, M., Feiner, C. & friedland, G. (1989) Risk factors for human immunodeficiency virus infection in intravenous drug users. *New England Journal of Medicine*, *321*, 874–879.

Schuckit, M. (1999) New findings in the genetics of alcoholism. *Journal of the American Medical Association*, *281*, 1875–1876.

Seal, K.H., Kral, A.H., Gee, L., Moore, L.D., Bluthenthal, R.N., Clorvick, J. & Edlin, B.R. (2001) Prediction and prevention of non-fatal overdose among street-recruited injection heroin users in the San Francisco Bay area, 1998–1999. *American Journal of Public Health*, *91*, 1842–1846.

Seal, K.H., Thawley, R., Gee, L., Bamberger, J., Kral, A.H., Ciccarone, D., Downing, M. & Edlin, B.R. (2005) Naloxone distribution and cardiopulmonary resuscitation training for injection drug users to prevent heroin overdose death: a pilot intervention. *Journal of Urban Health: Bulletin of the New York Academy of Medicine*, *82*, 303–311.

Seaman, S.R., Brettle, R.P. & Gore, S.M. (1998) Mortality from overdose among injecting drug users recently released from prison: database linkage study. *British Medical Journal*, *316*, 426–428.

Segest, E., Mygind, O. & Bay, H. (1990) The influence of prolonged stable methadone maintenance treatment on mortality and employment: an eight year follow-up. *International Journal of the Addictions*, *25*, 53–63.

Selim, V. & Kaplowitz, N. (1999) Hepatotoxicity of psychotropic drugs. *Hepatology*, 29, 1347–1351.

Seymour, A. & Oliver, J.S. (1999) Role of drugs and alcohol in impaired drivers and fatally injured drivers in the Strathclyde police region of Scotland, 1995–1998. *Forensic Science International*, 103, 89–100.

Seymour, A., Oliver, J.S. & Black, M. (2000) Drug-related deaths among recently released prisoners in the Strathclyde region of Scotland. *Journal of Forensic Sciences*, 45, 649–654.

Seymour, A., Black, M., Jay, J., Cooper, G., Weir, C. & Oliver, J. (2003) The role of methadone in drug-related deaths in the west of Scotland. *Addiction*, 98, 995–1002.

Shaffer, D., Gould, M.S., Fisher, P., Trautman, P., Moreau, D., Kleinman, M. & Flory, M. (1996) Psychiatric diagnosis in child and adolescent suicide. *Archives of General Psychiatry*, 53, 339–348.

Shaw, K.P. (1999) Human methamphetamine-related fatalities in Taiwan during 1991–1996. *Journal of Forensic Sciences*, 44, 27–31.

Sidney, S. (2002) Cardiovascular consequences of marijuana use. *Journal of Clinical Pharmacology*, 42, 64S–70S.

(2003) Comparing cannabis with tobacco – again – link between cannabis and mortality is still not established. *British Medical Journal*, 327, 635–636.

Sidney, S., Quesenberry, C.P., Friedman, G.D. & Tekawa, I.S. (1997) Marijuana use and cancer incidence (California, United States). *Cancer Causes and Control*, 8, 722–728.

Simini, B. (1998) Naloxone supplied to Italian heroin addicts. *Lancet*, 352, 967.

Simpson, D.D. & Sells, S.B. (1982) Effectiveness of treatment for drug abuse: an overview of the DARP research program. *Advances in Substance Abuse*, 2, 27–29.

Simpson, D.D., Joe, G.W. & Brown, B.S. (1997) Treatment retention and follow-up outcomes. The Drug Abuse Treatment Outcome Study (DATOS). *Psychology of Addictive Behaviors*, 4, 294–307.

Sjogren, H., Bjornstig, U., Eriksson, A., Ohman, U. & Solarz, A. (1997) Drug and alcohol use among injured motor vehicle drivers in Sweden: prevalence, driver, crash, and injury characteristics. *Alcoholism Clinical and Experimental Research*, 21, 968–973.

Spijkerman, I.J.B., Koot, M., Prins, M., Keet, I.P.M., Van den Hoek, A., Miedema, F. & Coutinho, R.A. (1995) Lower prevalence and incidence of HIV-1 syncytium-inducing phenotype among injecting drug users compared with homosexual men. *AIDS*, 9, 1085–1092.

Spirito, A., Brown, L., Overholser, J. & Fritz, G. (1989) Attempted suicide in adolescence: a review and critique of the literature. *Clinical Psychology Review*, 9, 335–363.

Spittal, P.M., Bruneau, J., Craib, K.J.P., Miller, C., Lamothe, F., Webber, A.E., Li, K., Tyndall, M.W., O'Shaughnessy, M.V. & Schechter, M.T. (2003) Surviving the sex trade: a comparison of HIV risk behaviours among street-involved women in two Canadian cities who inject drugs. *AIDS Care*, 15, 187–195.

Spunt, B., Goldstein, P., Brownstein, H., Fendrich, H. & Langley, S. (1994) Alcohol and homicide: interviews with prison inmates. *Journal of Drug Issues*, 24, 143–163.

Spunt, B., Goldstein, P., Brownstein, H., Fendrich, H. & Libertym H.J. (1995) Drug use by homicide offenders. *Journal of Psychoactive Drugs, 27*, 125–134.

Steentoft, A., Teige, B., Holmgren, P., Vuori, E., Kristinsson, J., Kaa, E., Wethe, G., Ceder, G., Pikkarainen, J. & Simonsen, K.W. (1996) Fatal poisonings in young drug addicts in the Nordic countries: a comparison between 1984–1985 and 1991, *Forensic Science International, 78*, 29–37.

Stefanis, C., Dornbush, R. & Fink, M. (1977) *Hashish: studies of long-term use.* New York: Raven Press.

Stewart, D., Gossop, M. & Marsden, J. (2002) Reductions in non-fatal overdose after drug misuse treatment: results from the National Treatment Outcome Research Study (NTORS). *Journal of Substance Abuse Treatment, 22*, 1–9.

Stimson, G. (1993) The global diffusion of injecting drug use: implications for human immunodeficiency virus infection. *Bulletin on Narcotics, 45*, 3–17.

Strain, E.C., Stitzer, M.L., Liebson, I.A. & Bigelow, G.E. (1994a) Buprenorphine versus methadone in the treatment of opioid-dependent cocaine users. *Psychopharmacology, 116*, 401–406.

(1994b) Comparison of buprenorphine and methadone in the treatment of opioid dependence. *American Journal of Psychiatry, 151*, 1025–1030.

Strang, J., Darke, S., Hall, W., Farrell, M. & Ali, R. (1996) Heroin overdose: Is there a case for take-home naloxone? *British Medical Journal, 312*, 1435.

Strang, J., Griffiths, P. & Gossop, M. (1997) Heroin smoking by "chasing the dragon": origins and history. *Addiction, 92*, 673–683.

Strang, J., Griffiths, P., Powis, B. & Gossop, M. (1999) Heroin chasers and heroin injectors: differences observed in a community sample in London, UK. *American Journal of the Addictions, 8*, 148–160.

Strang, J., Best, D., Man, L.H., Noble, A. & Gossop, M. (2000) Peer-initiated resuscitation: fellow drug users could be mobilised to implement resuscitation. *International Journal of Drug Policy, 11*, 437–445.

Strang, J., McCambridge, J., Best, D., Beswick, T., Bearn, J., Rees, S. & Gossop, M. (2003) Loss of tolerance and overdose mortality after inpatient opiate detoxification: follow up study. *British Medical Journal, 356*, 959–960.

Substance Abuse and Mental Health Services Administration (2005) *Results from the 2004 national survey on drug use and health: national findings.* Rockville, MD: Office of Applied Studies.

Suwaki, H. (1991) *Methamphetamine abuse in Japan. In M.A. Miller & N.J. Kozel (Eds), Methamphetamine abuse: epidemiologic issues and implications. NIDA research monograph no. 115 (pp. 84–98).* Rockville, MD: National Institute on Drug Abuse.

Sunjic, S. & Zador, D. (1999) Methadone related deaths in New South Wales 1990–1995. *Drug and Alcohol Review, 18*, 409–415.

Swalwell, C.I. & Davis, G.G. (1999) Methamphetamine as a risk factor for acute aortic dissection. *Journal of Forensic Sciences, 44*, 23–26.

Swift, W., Maher, L., Sunjic, S. & Doan, V. (1999) Transitions between routes of heroin administration: a study of Caucasian and Indochinese heroin users in South-western Sydney, Australia. *Addiction, 94,* 71–82.

Sztajnkrycer, M.D., Hariharan, S. & Bond, G.R. (2002) Cardiac irritability and myocardial infarction in a 13-year-old girl following recreational amphetamine overdose. *Pediatric Emergency Care, 18,* E11–E15.

Tagliaro, F., Debattisti, Z., Smith, F.P. & Marigo, M. (1998) Death from heroin overdose: findings from hair analysis. *Lancet, 351,* 1923–1925.

Tardiff, K., Marzuk, P.M., Leon, A., Portera, L., Hartwell, N., Hirsch, C.S. & Stajic, M. (1996) Accidental fatal drug overdoses in New York City: 1990–1992. *American Journal of Drug and Alcohol Abuse, 22,* 135–146.

Tardiff, K., Wallace, Z., Tracy, M., Piper, T.M., Vlahov, D. & Galea, S. (2005) Drug and alcohol use as determinants of New York City homicide trends from 1990 to 1998. *Journal of Forensic Sciences, 50,* 470–474.

Teesson, M., Havard, A., Fairbairn, S., Ross, J., Lynskey, M. & Darke, S. (2005) Depression among entrants to treatment for heroin dependence in the Australian Treatment Outcome Study (ATOS): prevalence, correlates and treatment seeking. *Drug and Alcohol Dependence, 78,* 309–315.

Teesson, M., Ross, J., Darke, S., Lynskey, M., Ali, R., Cooke, R. & Ritter, A. (2006) The Australian Treatment Outcome Study (ATOS): 1 year follow-up results. *Drug and Alcohol Dependence, 83,* 174–180.

Tennant, F.S. (1983) Clinical toxicology of cannabis use. In K. Fehr & H. Kalant (Eds), *Cannabis and Health Hazards.* Toronto, Ont.: Addiction Research Foundation.

Termorshuizen, F., Krol, A., Prins, M., van Ameijden, E.J.C. (2005) Long-term outcome of chronic drug use: The Amsterdam Cohort study among drug users. *American Journal of Epidemiology, 161,* 271–279.

Thiblin, I., Eksborg, S., Petersson, A., Fugelstad, A. & Rajs, J. (2004) Fatal intoxication as a consequence of intranasal administration (snorting) or pulmonary (smoking) of heroin. *Forensic Science International, 139,* 241–247.

Tien, P. (2005) Management and treatment of hepatitis C virus infection in HIV-infected adults: recommendations from the Veterans Affairs Hepatitis C Resource Center Program and National Hepatitis C Program Office. *American Journal of Gastroenterology, 100,* 2338–2354.

Tobler, N. & Stratton, H. (1997) Effectiveness of school-based drug prevention programs: a meta-analysis of the research. *Journal of Primary Prevention, 18,* 71–125.

Topp, L., Degenhardt, L., Kaye, S. & Darke, S. (2002) The emergence of potent forms of methamphetamine in Sydney, Australia; a case study of the IDRS as a strategic early warning system. *Drug and Alcohol Review, 21,* 341–348.

Topp, L., Day, C. & Degenhardt, L. (2003) Changes in patterns of drug injection concurrent with a sustained reduction in the availability of heroin in Australia. *Drug and Alcohol Dependence, 70,* 275–286.

Tortu, S., Neaigus, A., McMahon, J. & Hagen, D. (2001) Hepatitis C among noninjecting drug users: a report. *Substance Use & Misuse*, *36*, 523–534.

Tortu, S., McMahon, J.M., Pouget, E.R. & Hamid, R. (2004) Sharing of noninjection drug-use implements as a risk factor for hepatitis C. *Substance Use and Misuse*, *39*, 211–224.

Tracqui, A., Kintz, P. & Ludes, B. (1998) Buprenorphine-related deaths among drug addicts in France: a report on 20 fatalities. *Journal of Analytical Toxicology*, *22*, 430–434.

Tracy, M., Piper, T.M., Ompad, D., Bucciarelli, A., Coffin, P.O., Vlahov, D. & Galea, S. (2005) Circumstances of witnessed drug overdose in New York City: implications for intervention. *Drug and Alcohol Dependence*, *79*, 181–190.

Trull, T.J., Sher, K.J., Minks-Brown, C., Durbin, J. & Burr, R. (2000) Borderline personality disorder and substance use disorders: a review and integration. *Clinical Psychology Review*, *20*, 235–253.

Tsuang, M., Lyons, M., Eisen, S., Goldberg, J., True, W., Lin, N., Meyer, J., Toomey, R., Faraone, S. & Eaves, L. (1996) Genetic influences on DSM-III-R drug abuse and dependence: a study of 3 372 twin pairs. *American Journal of Medical Genetics (Neuropsychiatric Genetics)*, *67*, 473–477.

Tsuang, M.T., Lyons, M.J., Meyer, J.M., Doyle, T., Eisen, S.A., Goldberg, J., True, W., Lin, N., Toomey, R. & Eaves, L. (1998) Co-occurrence of abuse of different drugs in men: the role of drug-specific and shared vulnerabilities [see comments]. *Archives of General Psychiatry*, *55*, 967–972.

Tuan, N.A., Hien, N.T., Chi, P.K., Giang, L.T., Thang, B., Long, H., Saidel, T. & Roger, M. (2004) Intravenous drug use among street-based sex workers: a high-risk behaviour for HIV transmission. *Sexually Transmitted Diseases*, *31*, 15–19.

Tunkel, A.R. & Pradhan, S.K. (2002) Central nervous system infections in injection drug users. *Infectious Disease Clinics of North America*, *16*, 589–605.

Tunving, K. (1988) Fatal outcome in drug addiction. *Acta Psychiatrica Scandinavia*, *77*, 551–566.

Turk, E.E. & Tsokos, M. (2004) Pathologic features of fatal falls from height. *American Journal of Forensic Medicine and Pathology*, *25*, 194–199.

Turnipseed, S.D., Richards, J.R., Kirk, J.D., Diercks, D.B. & Amsterdam, E.A. (2003) Frequency of acute coronary syndrome in patients presenting to the emergency department with chest pain after methamphetamine use. *Journal of Emergency Medicine*, *24*, 369–373.

Tyndall, M.W., Craib, K.J.P., Currie, S., Li, K., O'Shaughnessy, M.V. & Schechter, M.T. (2001) Impact of HIV infection on mortality in a cohort of injection drug users. *Journal of Acquired Immune Deficiency Syndromes*, *28*, 351–357.

Umbricht, A., Hoover, D.R., Tucker, M.J., Leslie, J.M., Chaisson, R.E. & Preston, K.L. (2003) Opioid detoxification with buprenorphine, clonidine, or methadone in hospitalized heroin-dependent patients with HIV infection. *Drug and Alcohol Dependence*, *69*, 263–272.

UNAIDS (2002) *Report on the global HIV/AIDS epidemic 2002.* Retrieved, 2004, from the World Wide Web: http://www.unaids.org.

 (2004) *2004 Report on the global AIDS epidemic. 4th global report.* Geneva: UNAIDS/04.16E.

United Nations Drug Control Programme (2000) *Global illicit drug trends 2000.* Vienna: United Nations Drug Control Programme.

United Nations Office for Drug Control (2004) *World illict drug report 2004.* New York: United Nations Publications.

 (2005) *World illict drug report 2005.* New York: United Nations Publications.

Urbina, A. & Jones, K. (2004) Crystal methamphetamine, its analogues, and HIV infection: medical and psychiatric aspects of a new epidemic. *Clinical Infectious Diseases, 38*, 890–894.

Vaillant, G. (1973) A 20 year follow–up of New York narcotic addicts. *Archives of General Psychiatry, 29*, 237–241.

Valenciano, M., Emmanuelli, J. & Lert, F. (2001) Unsafe injecting practices among attendees of syringe exchange programmes in France. *Addiction, 96*, 597–606.

Van Ameijden, E.J.C., Krol, A., Vlahov, D., Flynn, C., van Haarstrecht, H.J.A. & Coutinho, R.A. (1999a) Pre-AIDS mortality and morbidity among injection drug users in Amsterdam and Baltimore: an ecological comparison. *Substance Use and Misuse, 34*, 845–865.

van Ameijden, E.J.C., Langemdazm, M.W. & Coutinho, R.A. (1999b) Dose-effect relationship between overdose mortality and prescribed methadone dosage in low-threshold maintenance programs. *Addictive Behaviors, 24*, 559–563.

Van Haarstrecht, H.J.A., van Ameijden, E.J.C., van den Hoek, J.A.R., Mientjes, G.H.C., Bax, J.S. & Coutinho, R.A. (1996) Predictors of mortality in the Amsterdam cohort of human immunodeficiency virus (HIV)-positive and HIV-negative drug users. *American Journal of Epidemiology, 143*, 380–391.{net}

Vasica, G. & Tennant, C.C. (2002) Cocaine use and cardiovascular complications. *Medical Journal of Australia, 177*, 260–262.

Velleman, R., Templeton, L. & Copello, A. (2005) The role of the family in preventing and intervening with substance use and misuse: a comprehensive review of family interventions, with a focus on young people. *Drug and Alcohol Review, 24*, 93–109.

Vimpani, G. (2005) Getting the mix right: family, community and social policy interventions to improve outcomes for young people at risk of substance misuse. *Drug and Alcohol Review, 24*, 111–125.

Vingoe, L., Welch, S., Farrell, M. & Strang, J. (1999) Heroin overdose among a treatment sample of injecting drug misusers: accident or suicidal behaviour? *Journal of Substance Use, 4*, 88–91.

Vlahov, D. & Junge, B. (1998) The role of needle exchange programs in HIV prevention. *Public Health Reports, 113*(Suppl 1), 75–80.

Vlahov, D., Wang, C., Galai, N., Bareta, J., Mehta, S.H., Strathdee, S.A. & Nelson, K.E. (2004) Mortality risk among new onset injection drug users. *Addiction, 99*, 946–954.

Vlahov, D., Galai, N., Safaeian, M., Galea, S., Kirk, G., Lucas, G.M. & Sterling, T.R. (2005) Effectiveness of highly active antiretroviral therapy among injection drug users with late-stage human immunodeficiency virus infection. *American Journal of Epidemiology*, *161*, 999–1012.

Wahren, C.A., Brandt, L. & Allebeck, P. (1997) Has mortality in drug addicts increased? A comparison between hospitalized cohorts in Stockholm. *International Journal of Epidemiology*, *26*, 1219–1226.

Waksman, J., Taylor, R.N., Bodor, G.S., Daly, F.F.S., Jolliff, H.A. & Dart, R.C. (2001) Acute myocardial infarction associated with methamphetamine use. *Mayo Clinic Proceedings*, *76*, 323–326.

Walker, D.J., Zacny, J.P., Galva, K.E. & Lichtor, J.L. (2001) Subjective, psychomotor, and physiological effects of cumulative doses of mixed-action opioids in health volunteers. *Psychopharmacology*, *155*, 362–371.

Walsh, J.M., de Gier, J.J., Christopherson, A.S. & Verstraete, A.G. (2004) Drugs and driving. *Traffic Injury Prevention*, *5*, 241–253.

Ward, J., Mattick, R.P. & Hall, W. (1992) *Key issues in methadone maintenance treatment*. Sydney: New South Wales University Press.

(1998) *Methadone maintenance treatment and other opioid replacement therapies*. Amsterdam: Harwood.

Ward, J., Hall, W. & Mattick, R.P. (1999) Role of maintenance treatment in opioid dependence. *Lancet*, *353*, 221–226.

Warner, L.A., Kessler, R.C., Hughes, M., Anthony, J.C. & Nelson, C.B. (1995) Prevalence and correlates of drug use and dependence in the United States. Results from the National Comorbidity Survey. *Archives of General Psychiatry*, *52*, 219–229.

Warner-Smith, M., Darke, S., Lynskey, M. & Hall, W. (2001) Heroin overdose: causes and consequences. *Addiction*, *96*, 1113–1125.

Warner-Smith, M., Darke, S. & Day, C. (2002) Morbidity associated with non-fatal heroin overdose. *Addiction*, *97*, 963–967.

Watterson, O., Simpson, D.W. & Sells, S.B. (1975) Death rates and causes of death among opioid addicts in community drug treatment programs during 1970–1973. *American Journal of Drug and Alcohol Abuse*, *2*, 99–111.

Webb, L., Oyefesso, A., Schifano, F., Cheeta, S., Pollard, M. & Ghodse, A.H. (2003) Cause and manner of death in drug-related fatality: an analysis of drug-related deaths recorded by coroners in England and Wales in 2000. *Drug and Alcohol Dependence*, *72*, 67–74.

Welder, A.A. (1992) A primary culture system of postnatal rat heart cells for the study of cocaine and methamphetamine toxicity. *Toxicology Letters*, *60*, 183–196.

Wetli, C.V. & Wright, R.K. (1979) Death caused by recreational cocaine use. *JAMA*, *241*, 2519–2522.

White, D. & Pitts, P. (1998) Educating young people about drugs: a systematic review. *Addiction*, *93*, 1475–1487.

White, J. & Irvine, R. (1999) Mechanisms of fatal opioid overdose. *Addiction*, *95*, 961–972.

Wijetunga, M., Seto, T., Lindsay, J. & Schatz, I. (2003) Crystal methamphetamine-associated cardiomyopathy: tip of the iceberg? *Journal of Toxicology – Clinical Toxicology, 41*, 981–986.

Weatherburn, D. & Lind, B. (2001) *Delinquent-Prone Communities.* Cambridge: Cambridge University Press.

Wilkins, C. (2002) Designer amphetamines in New Zealand: policy challenges and initiatives. *Social Policy Journal of New Zealand, 19*, 14–27.

Wilkinson, R. & Marmot, M. (Eds) (2003) *The solid facts: social determinants of health (2nd Edition).* Copenhagen: Centre for Urban Health World Health Organization.

Wille, R. (1981) Ten-year follow-up of a representative sample of London heroin addicts: attendance, abstinence and mortality. *British Journal of Addiction, 76*, 259–266.

Williamson, P.A., Foreman, K.J., White, J.M. & Anderson, G. (1997) Methadone-related overdose deaths in South Australia, 1984–1994. How safe is prescribing? *Medical Journal of Australia, 166*, 302–305.

Wodak, A. & Lurie, P. (1996) A tale of two countries: attempting to control HIV among injecting drug users in Australia and the United States. *Journal of Drug Issues, 27*, 117–134.

World Health Organization (1993) *The ICD-10 classification of mental and behavioural disorders.* Vienna: World Health Organization.

Zaccarelli, M., Gattari, P., Rezza, G., Conti, S., Spizzichino, L., Vlahov, D., Ippolito, G., Lelli, V. & Valenza, C. (1994) Impact of HIV infection on non-AIDS mortality among Italian injecting drug users. *AIDS, 8*, 345–350.

Zador, D. & Sunjic, S. (2000) Deaths in methadone maintenance treatment in New South Wales, Australia 1990–1995. *Addiction, 95*, 77–84.

(2002) Methadone-related deaths and mortality rate during induction into methadone maintenance, New South Wales, 1996. *Drug and Alcohol Review, 21*, 131–136.

Zanis, D.A. & Woody, G.E. (1998) One-year mortality rates following methadone treatment discharge. *Drug and Alcohol Dependence, 52*, 257–260.

Zhu, B.L., Oritani, S., Shimotouge, K., Ishida, K., Quan, L., Fujita, M.Q., Ogawa, M. & Maeda, H. (2000) Methamphetamine-related fatalities in forensic autopsy during 5 years in the southern half of Osaka city and surrounding areas. *Forensic Sciences International, 113*, 443–447.

Index

Note: Page numbers in *italics* refer to tables.